# Healing

# You

Teresa Cody

# DEDICATION

This book is dedicated to my mother, Doris, and my grandmother, Margaret, who were both highly influential in teaching me about vitamins and whole non-processed organic foods at a time when no one else was thinking about those ideas. It led to my love of natural healing and natural healing modalities.

# ACKNOWLEDGMENTS

There are many people to thank who trusted me to "try" this treatment on them with little reservation. To my good friend, Tara Murski, who believed my scientific theory and allowed herself to be the first guinea pig. I am forever in your debt.

Thank you, Charles Runels M.D., for training and supporting medical providers with your focus on platelet rich plasma.

Thank you, Glenna Scott R.N., for jumping into this adventure without hesitation and bringing smart ideas to the treatments of all the patients.

Thank you, George Miller M.D., for supporting the wellness center and the ideas of using natural healing modalities.

Lastly, I want to thank my husband, Timothy Cashion, for always encouraging me to try new things and supporting me.

# TABLE OF CONTENTS

# INTRODUCTION

Why write this book?

For me, this is the easiest question to answer! For the past two years, I have seen miracles happen, and I want to share these miracles with everyone in the world.

Through every blood vessel inside of you, the miracle courses and it is waiting to activate itself when needed. How do you activate this glorious golden liquid? Injure yourself and the miracle jumps to attention and heals the injury without being asked.

It is the healing power inside every animal. This miracle is you healing you! The reason it works so well is that God made it, not man.

The reason for this book is to inform you of one excellent and safe alternative treatment that may help you heal an injury. It is so important that you learn about Platelet Rich Plasma (PRP) and keep it in your back pocket in case you need a miracle. This book will show you one miracle after another.

Platelet Rich Plasma (PRP) therapy uses injections as a concentrate of a patient's own platelets, plasma and healing factors to speed up the repair of injured tendons, ligaments, muscles and joints. In this way, PRP injections use each individual patient's own healing system to improve musculoskeletal problems and much more as you will soon see.

Vampire Facial® uses PRP for esthetics facial rejuvenation. It has become popular across the US because several celebrities tout the gorgeous effects of your own healing factors. But PRP is also used for many other conditions. In this book, I present our clinical observations and our experience using PRP in many conditions.

To share this information with every person in the world is my goal. Everyone should understand how you can heal yourself with a safe treatment that is therapeutic. You will soon see how scars disappear, diabetic sores and ulcerations heal, plantar fasciitis resolves eliminating foot pain, trigger fingers calm down, tendon and ligaments repair themselves, and on the esthetic side, skin glows with beautiful health and much more.

# CHAPTER 1:
# MY JOURNEY INTO PRP

I have such gratitude for the information I received about Platelet Rich Plasma (PRP). My journey began with my hairdresser, Tara. She has been a hairdresser for 37 years (yeah, if you saw her you would ask—did she start at five years old?). Tara hurt her right hand from the repetitive motion of drying hair. It's the motion of rolling the hair on to a round brush and pulling the hair horizontally. The motion none of us can do to ourselves at home. This is the reason our hair never looks as good as the day we go to the hairdresser. The poor girls in those blow dry bars! All day, every day, the same repetitive motion! They will find out that the body hates repetitive motions.

We all understand the repetitive motion of drying hair but she learned to cut hair using her ring finger doing all the scissor motion and keeping her thumb stationary. Her ring finger was a major trigger finger!

Her thumb and fingers could no longer touch. She could not make a fist. Six months before, she had received a steroid shot, and her pain disappeared for four months and four days. She was heading to get another steroid shot and something made me blurt out—"No, let's try PRP first."

She asked, "What's that?"

This was the start of a wonderful journey.

Platelet Rich Plasma or PRP for short is the healing portion of the blood. It contains healing factors and much more.

Dentistry has embraced the use of PRP since the early 1990s [1]. I remember the oral surgeon in our building, showing my husband and I his new centrifuge, with great excitement. Bone grafting in the jawbone is unsuccessful without PRP and without bone there is no way to restore a lost tooth with a dental implant. For 30 years, professionals have used PRP in dentistry without adverse side effects.

Platelet Rich Plasma (PRP) is defined as an autologous treatment because it derives from an individual and transfers into the same individual. There is no donor. It is "you" healing "you" with healing growth factors in your own blood!

When you skin your knee, the healing happens because of PRP. It clots the scrape, produces the scab and starts healing, plus it has antibacterial immune cells. Remember, dentists have used PRP since the early 1990s for bone grafts, but what is so strange is that I had never used it in my dental practice. The surgeon in our office does. I don't even know why I thought of it and blurted it out. It was a gift from God.

Tara and I have been friends for many years. She takes care of my hair and I take care of her Botox and dermal filler and teeth. She has been a patient for many years. After explaining to Tara what PRP is and that the worst that could happen was that it did nothing to help her, she agreed to try PRP. She did not tell me if she was apprehensive, however, I know she was desperate to ease the pain. I think she trusted me because concentrating on your own healing factors makes sense.

The next Monday afternoon, she came to my dental office, and I explained that we would draw blood, run it through the centrifuge, pipette off the top layer of PRP and inject the yellow PRP into the damaged areas. At the last minute I said, "Let's take a picture." Thank God I did. No one would believe what happened in the next two days.

Figure 1: Tara's pretreatment fist

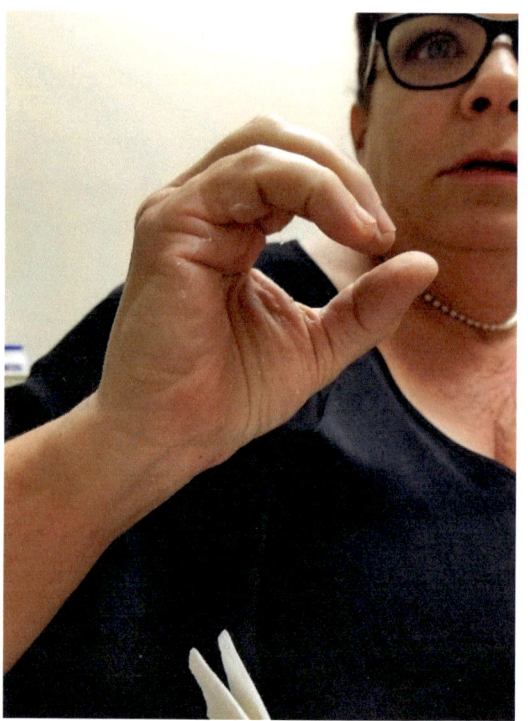

Here is the before picture of her trying to make a fist. She could not even come close to making a fist. The picture illustrates the damage to her digital dexterity.

We drew one test tube of her blood, ran it through the centrifuge, and injected it under the skin into her hand which houses the repetitive motion damage. She asked when she would notice any changes. I did not know what we would see. "Maybe six weeks," I said. The only reference point I had was that after a dental bone graft we wait three months to place a dental implant.

Figure 2: Tara's fist 12 hours after PRP treatment

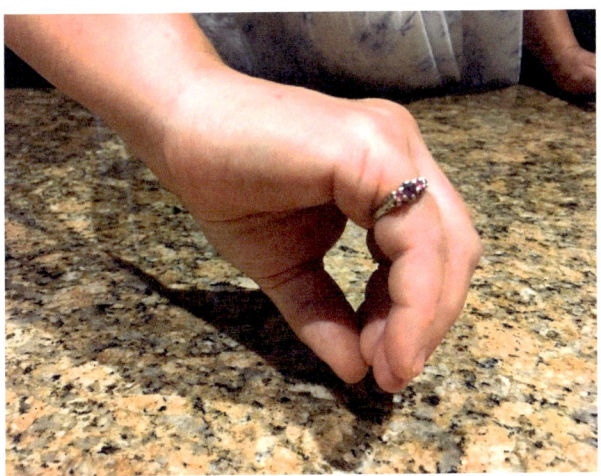

The next morning, I received a text from her. Her fingers and thumb now touched each other. What? In 12 hours?

But I never expected the photo she texted the next day! I injected her Monday afternoon and by Wednesday she sent this photo of a fantastic full-fledged fist.

Figure 3: Tara's fist 2 days after PRP treatment

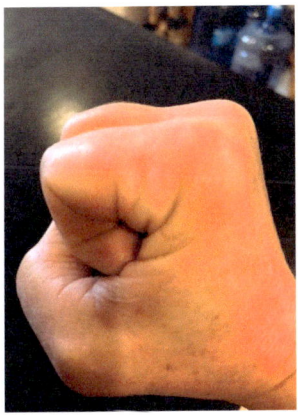

In two days, she could make a fist! Now I am intrigued! This is the most exciting development I have ever seen.

What is this magical golden fluid inside of all of us? How does it work? With every spare minute, I read everything about PRP I could get my hands on (and with the Internet that was a LOT). I retired from dentistry, but PRP lured me out of retirement with its ability to heal, create beauty, and decrease pain. PRP has at least 15 healing factors and antimicrobial factors.[2] God knew when we skinned our knees, we would need protection from E. coli and Staph.

References for Chapter 1:

1.  Anitua, E. (1999). Plasma rich in growth factors: preliminary results of use in the preparation of future sites for implants. *The International journal of oral & maxillofacial implants,* 14(4), 529-35. PMID: 10453668

2.  Pavlovic, V., Ciric, M., Jovanovic, V., & Stojanovic, P. (2016). Platelet Rich Plasma: a short overview of certain bioactive components. *Open medicine (Warsaw, Poland),* 11(1), 242-7. PMID: 28352802 PMCID: PMC5329835 DOI: 10.1515/med-2016-0048

.

# CHAPTER 2:
# SYNCHRONICITY

S ome people call it synchronicity. Some people call it serendipity. I call it the actions of God. After seeing the remarkable changes with her hand, I knew I would have to investigate Platelet Rich Plasma (PRP) further.

October 1, 2018, is the day that changed my calling. That is the day I injected PRP into Tara's hand. Within two weeks, we got a call from our tenant asking to get out of her lease six months early. We have 1900 square feet built out for a med-spa next to our dental office. It has six treatment rooms ready to see patients. My first thought was to get another tenant, but within two weeks I thought maybe I should open a wellness center. My husband and I talked about it and debated it. We weighed all the pros and cons. My husband said, "Why don't you try for a year? If it doesn't work out, we can always lease the space."

"Okay, let's go for it!"

As I scoured the internet for every article on PRP, I ran into the Vampire Facial®. What could PRP do for aging skin and wrinkles? If it healed the face like it did Tara's hand, this would be an aesthetic breakthrough.

I took the next available course on PRP and facial esthetics, called the Vampire Facelift® with Dr. Charles Runels, the inventor, in Fairhope, Alabama.

I wanted to learn from the inventor and learn from the best. It was a great course with live models to practice on. Within 24 hours, the live models had a beautiful glow on their faces. I kept staring and my skin seemed sooo dull. I couldn't wait to get this glorious procedure going in my new office.

The changes we have seen with the facial skin are outstanding! The skin glows! With all those healing factors in the PRP, the damaged and aged skin heals and becomes more youthful. The pores close, wrinkles smooth out, and the skin becomes vibrant and glowing.

Now I have a place where I can treat patients, but I am a dentist and I needed a nurse to draw blood. I did not know how to do that yet. Where was I going to get a nurse?

In November, I had a quilting course at my house for about six women. One of them was a retired nurse. As soon as Glenna walked through the door, I asked her if she would like to work with me. She did not even hesitate for a second. "Absolutely!" was her response.

See, I told you, the universe worked fast! Every time I turned around, another door opened.

I tried to open on a shoestring budget, but when I showed Glenna the space the colors disturbed her. Some countertops were a lime green plastic that tried to imitate glass countertops with gold cabinets. Do you remember the color blocking fad? One blue wall, a dark green wall combined with purple columns. This was NOT a soothing, comfortable space.

We had to paint. We not only had to paint some walls, we had to paint some countertops and Formica cabinets. I went to a big box store and a guy in the paint department was the best. He showed me everything

I needed to get the paint to stick to Formica and plastic countertops. I had no budget to rip out the cabinets and replace them.

The countertop paint stuck, but not without damaging some brain cells along the way. Whew, that paint smelled strong but did its job and camouflaged the lime green plastic countertops.

The place needed a scrub down too. After a few weeks, it looked great. New furniture was a must and some lovely decorations helped soften the whole look. Now, people comment on how nice the office is. We are one step closer to opening in what became a fantastic journey.

We are almost ready to open our doors, but Glenna and I wanted to make sure we were ready for prime time. I began recruiting my employees for Vampire Facial®. Glenna and I had to develop the flow of the procedures.

Glenna has had a stellar nursing career starting in the trauma ICU unit then making her way into research, which she loved. She worked studies looking at stem cell procedures before they became mainstream. PRP is right up her alley.

Glenna and I met through my sister, Cynthia, which was another act of the universe. My sister invited me to the Houston Quilt Festival, which is the largest quilt festival in the world. But here's the rub. I don't quilt or at least didn't. I went because they have rows and rows of shopping! Then we went antique shopping at a Texas tradition called Antiques Weekend in Warrenton, Texas.

This "weekend" is three weeks in duration. It stretches for 10 miles and is field after field of antique vendors. It's mind boggling how many people gather here twice a year. I have gone for at least 20 years and I don't want to miss it. You might stumble upon the perfect treasure.

The day before we went antiquing Cynthia called and canceled. Glenna texted, "I guess we are not going." I texted back, "I still want to go." We spent the day together shopping for junk and antiques, walking for miles and miles through the fields of Warrenton, TX. We had a blast, and we connected. Now, here we are starting a new business.

We quickly learned that we make a great team. Our backgrounds are vastly different so together we have many diverse ideas. I love that we can collaborate and bounce ideas off of each other.

At first, we offered a Vampire Facial®. to every employee and close friends. The results were superb. Within a week of receiving the Vampire Facial®, each employee's skin looked better and better. We observed large pores become smaller. One employee's melasma (dark areas on the skin) lightening. One of the best descriptions is the skin has a distinctive glow to it. The skin looks better than I have ever seen using any other product! Here are some before and after pictures.

Figure 4: Before and After 4 Vampire Facials®

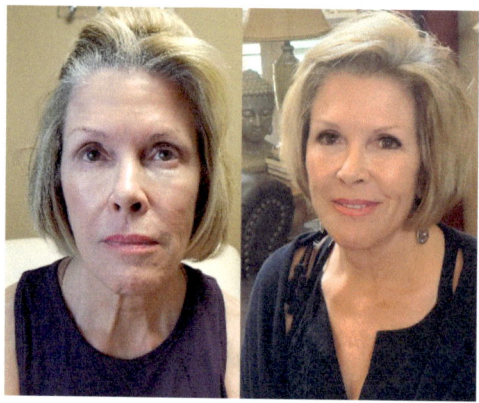

Meet Julie, notice all "freckles" [sun spots] have disappeared. Both pictures were taken without any foundation makeup.

Figure 5: Before and After 3 Vampire Facials®

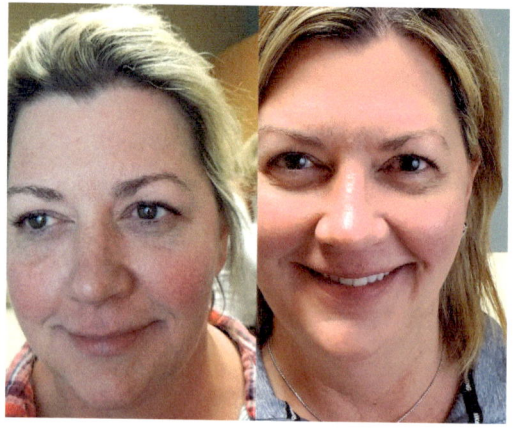

Meet Janus, her skin has improved texture and color after one Vampire Facial®. She looks vibrant and her skin glows.

Figure 6: Before and After 1 Vampire Facial®

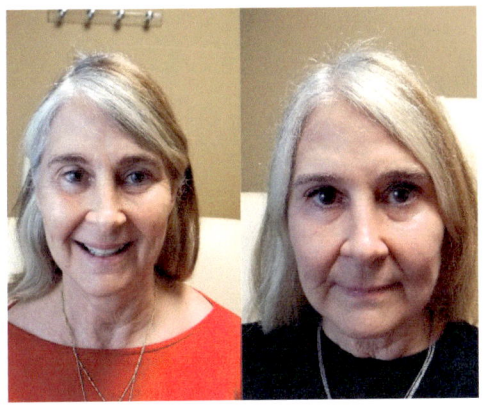

Meet Laela, her face looks great, but she was thrilled with the response of the skin on her neck.

Figure 7: Before and After 1 PRP neck treatment

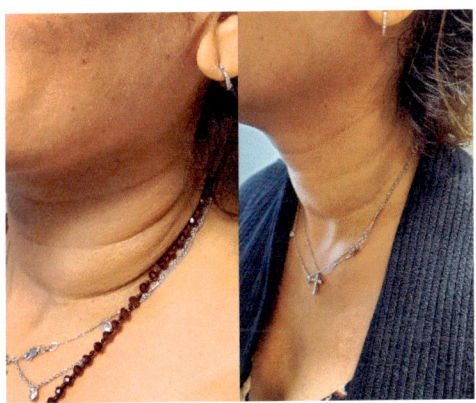

Meet Mattie, another example of vibrant, glowing skin. She is adorable.

Figure 8: Before and After 1 Vampire Facial®

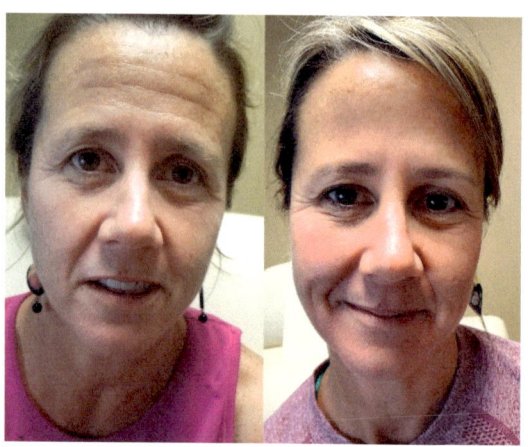

Meet Sherri, one of my dental assistants who has been fighting melasma which are brown spots. She has tried many treatments, including chemical peels, whitening creams, to name a few. Her melasma almost completely disappeared after only 2 Vampire Facials®

Figure 9: Before and After 2 Vampire Facial®

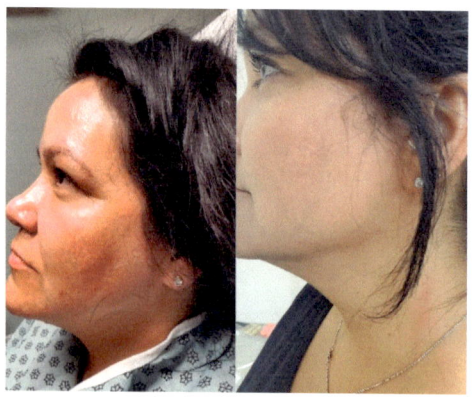

Meet Kathy, her natural beauty is enhanced with the Vampire Facial®

Figure 10: Before and After 3 Vampire Facials®

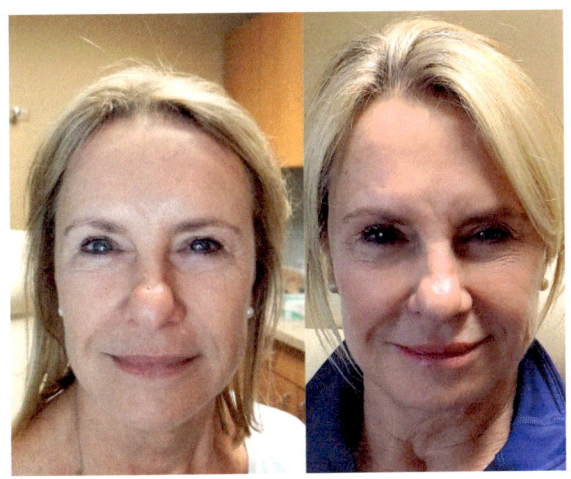

One of the first amazing results we saw was with Glenna's son, Stanley. Stanley had a dog that was a little nervous, to put it mildly. His sister, a professional dog trainer, told him to get rid of the dog. She said the dog was neurotic and untrainable. Did he listen? Ugh, no.

One day he startled this neurotic dog, and the dog bit him on the face. On his nose. He went to the ER but they cannot close up a dog bite because of fear of bacterial infection. The bite was in the shape of a "z."

Here is a picture of the severe bite:

Figure 11: Stanley in the hospital the day of the dog bite

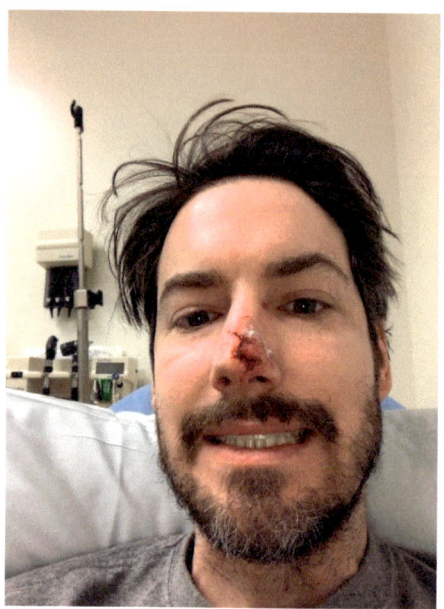

Eight weeks later he was in town for business and we injected PRP around the prominent scar. It was not only red but raised at least 1/8th of an inch.

Figure 12: Before PRP treatment

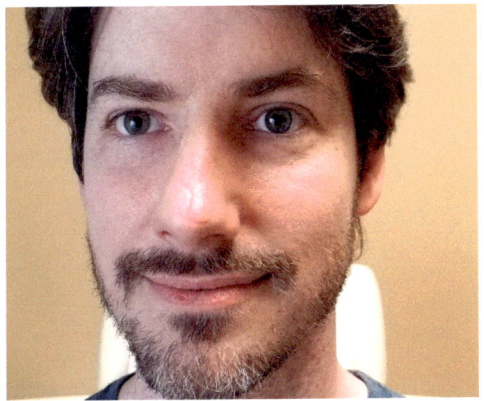

Since he lives out of town, we did not see him again in the office for 12 weeks. Here are the results from one treatment of PRP in a fresh scar. It disappeared, and the raised portion of the scar levelled out. The scar disappeared and you can see his skin is glowing.

Figure 13: After 1 PRP treatment

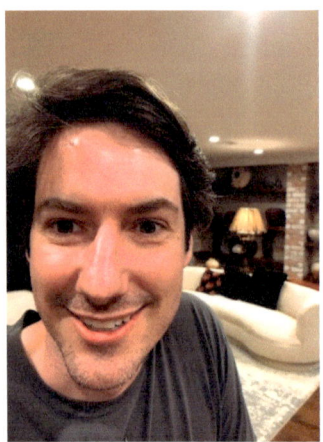

Where is the scar?

Glenna's family continued to give us problems to treat with PRP. Her son-in-law, Ion, tore a tendon in his second toe while he was running. You know how it is, trying to get in shape and you hurt something else. He went to an MD who offered three viable treatments: Surgery to shorten the second toe; Stem cell injection; or PRP injection.

The research using PRP and PRP plus stem cells on torn tendons and ligaments started less than 20 years ago. Tendons are tough bands of fibrous connective tissue that attach muscle to bone. As you contract the muscle, the tendon stabilizes the motion and tendons also have a spring action so they need to bounce with elasticity to the muscle action. Not all studies showed significant healing at 14 days post treatment, comparing a PRP group and a control group (researchers use saline for the control group). However, when they measured the strength of the tendon, there was a significant increase in the mechanical strength, and the elasticity of the healed tendon [1]. Later studies showed that PRP can speed up early phase inflammation leading to faster tendon repair and tendon strength [2]; It also increases the tendon's ability to handle use quicker therefore, faster recovery from an injury and quicker ability to get back in the game. This might be the reason professional sports organizations have used PRP for a long time. Those players are worth a lot of money and must get back in the game as soon as possible.

In 2008, Kajikawa et al., showed that PRP increased blood flow at the site of the injection which helps to bring necessary cells to begin the healing process [3]. They also showed that the body used collagen type 1 when they injected PRP in the area as opposed to type 3 collagen, which has a weaker biomechanical profile leading to more relapses. All these reasons and the safety of injecting autologous PRP seemed like a simple decision. We decided we might as well try to see if we could heal the ripped tendon.

Ion's second toe leaned on the big toe. He could not lift it and he had constant pain. We numbed the toe and injected 2 ccs into the area of the torn tendon. I wondered if the tendon would heal properly if we did not somehow brace the toe. His MD prescribed a toe brace to correct the hurt toe's position which the patient wore for the next eight weeks.

We did not take before photos, but within eight weeks, the pain disappeared, and he had full use of the toe. Here is a photo of him being able to lift the toe.

Figure 14: After 1 PRP treatment

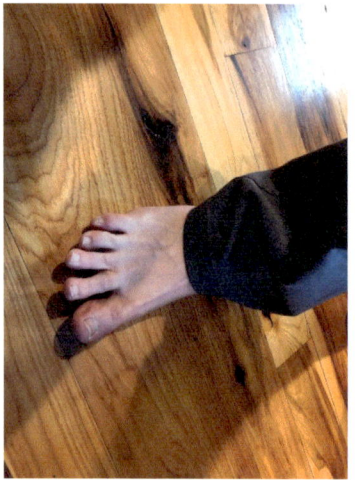

Another study looked at tendon stem cells and the effects PRP had on them. PRP activated tendon stem cells contributing to the quick healing of the treated tendon [4].

We went head to toe with PRP. Our eyes opened to the possibilities. The body uses PRP to heal. Let's look at what is in this miracle that courses through all your blood vessels.

References for Chapter 2:

1.  Molloy T, Wang Y, Murrell AC. 2003; The roles of Growth
    Factors in tendon healing and ligament healing. Sports Med
    33(5):381-394 PMID: 12696985 DOI: 10.2165/00007256-
    200333050-00004

2.  Aspenberg P, Virchenko O. (2004) Platelet concentrate
    injection improves Achilles tendon repair in rats. Acta
    Orthopaed Scand 75(1):93-99 PMID: 15022816
    DOI: 10.1080/00016470410001708190

3.  Kajikawa Y, Morihara T, Sakamoto H et al.(2008) Platelet
    Rich Plasma enhances the initial mobilization of circulation
    derived cells for tendon healing. J Cell Physiol 215(3):837-845
    PMID: 18181148 DOI: 10.1002/jcp.21368

4.  Zhang J, Nie D, Williamson K, et al. (2019) Selectively
    activated PRP exerts differential effects on tendon stem
    /progenitor cells and tendon healing. J Tissue Eng Jan.–Dec.
    PMID: 30728936 PMCID: PMC6351965
    DOI: 10.1177/2041731418820034

# CHAPTER 3:
# THE MIRACLE INSIDE YOUR BODY

In the mid 1990s, I read a study about stem cells. The researchers knew that stem cells could help spinal cord injuries, but they did not know how they could deliver them to the exact location of the trauma. They injected a mouse with tagged stem cells distant from the trauma. To the researchers' amazement, the stem cells migrated to the exact location of the trauma and began their job. Healing the damage! The body is a miracle. We have observed this same phenomenon with the healing factors in PRP.

We all have stem cells. Adult stem cells are undifferentiated cells found throughout the body that divide to replenish dying cells and regenerate damaged tissues. We can find them throughout the body. These cells can transform into any cell your body needs—acting as part of the repair system for the body.

There are three accessible sources of your own stem cells:

1. Bone Marrow

2. Adipose tissue (fat cells)

3. Blood

Extracting stem cells from bone marrow requires drilling into bone and harvesting the stem cells. They often come from the thigh bone or hip bone.

They also extract stem cells from fat tissue. There is a special centrifuge that can extract your stem cells from your fat cells in about one hour. But don't get too excited about shedding a bunch of fat; it only requires about 30 cc (ml) which is not much.

Option three to access your stem cells is through your blood. Blood runs through a machine and it separates the stem cells from the other blood components.

Collected and "minimally manipulated" stem cells are FDA approved. This means no one can grow them in a petri dish and then re-implant them.

A simple way to get stem cells to the site of the injury is to attract them using PRP (Platelet Rich Plasma) which is available in your blood. We have known for some time that the platelet portion of the blood is essential to the healing process. At first, we recognized it as the clotting portion of the blood. We now know it also has other functions like inflammation, healing, immunity, and tissue regeneration. These tiny blood components are loaded with growth factors, antimicrobial factors, and tissue regenerative factors.

For example, let's say you skin your knee. Platelets will ooze into the wound and start the clotting process. At the same time, it releases anti-microbial factors that kill any bacterial infection, then the growth factors kick into gear and direct the healing process whereby the tissue regenerates itself. This is miraculous!

The growth factors are also time released so that they work over a week or more. They attract stem cells and direct new blood vessels to form. With new blood vessels, more blood flows to the injury, bringing more healing factors to the area. The growth factors also stimulate collagen to form and they enhance tissue proliferation and regeneration.

PRP is readily available with a simple blood draw. We spin the drawn blood in a centrifuge. The red blood cells are heavier than platelets, so they sink to the bottom of the test tube. The platelets and plasma float on top of the red blood cells. We pipette off the platelets, the plasma and all those beautiful growth factors.

PRP is an excellent resource to concentrate on healing in a specific area. It can boost healing into high gear. Have you ever fed fish in an aquarium? Those fish swim to the surface and gobble down the food. Imagine, your cells are the little fish and the PRP is the food. Your body gobbles up the PRP and loves the growth factors.

**Growth Factors**

A growth factor is a naturally occurring substance capable of stimulating cell growth, proliferation, healing, and cellular differentiation. Growth factors are proteins and hormones, and they are super important for cellular function and healing.

Growth factors act as leaders of the cells. Telling the undifferentiated cell "OK, now you need to become a skin cell." They do this by binding on the outside of the cell on specific receptors. The cell responds to the growth factor by following the specific instructions.

Growth factors lead the way with many instructions. To give you an idea, scan the list below. The best part is we have access to them all the time. They are part of your circulating blood all the time.

Here is a list of growth factors and their jobs:

• platelet-derived growth factor (PDGF) It regulates and triggers cell growth and cell division. PDGF plays a substantial role in blood vessel formation and the growth of blood vessels from already existing blood vessel tissue [1].

• transforming growth factor beta (TGF-Beta) Some of its role in healing is to regulate the inflammation process. It has a crucial role in differentiation of stem cells and it directs stem cells to become a specific cell. There is still much to learn about this growth factor and all the growth factors [2].

• fibroblast growth factor (FGF) are multifunctional proteins with a wide variety of effects; they stimulate cell division but also have regulatory, morphological, and endocrine (hormone) effects. We sometimes call them "promiscuous" growth factors because of their multiple actions on multiple cell types. In healing, they stimulate blood vessel formation, skin growth, and fibroblasts to proliferate and give rise to tissue, which fills up a wound space early in the wound-healing process) [3].

• FGFs are also important for maintenance of the adult brain. They are major factors of neuronal survival and during adulthood. Adult neurogenesis (growing new nerves in the brain) within the hippocampus (area in brain involved with learning and memory) [4].

• insulin-like growth factor 1 (IGF-1) has growth-promoting effects on almost every cell in the body, including skeletal muscle, cartilage, bone, liver, kidney, nerve, skin, blood cells, and lung cells. IGF-1 can also regulate cellular DNA synthesis [5]

• insulin-like growth factor 2 (IGF-2) Circulates in the blood and regulates growth [6]

• vascular endothelial growth factor (VEGF)is a signal protein that helps to form blood vessels. It is part of the system that restores the oxygen supply to tissues when blood circulation is inadequate, such as in hypoxic conditions[7]. VEGF's normal function is to create new blood vessels during embryonic development, new blood vessels after injury, muscle following exercise, and new vessels (collateral circulation) to bypass blocked vessels.

• epidermal growth factor (EGF) results in cellular proliferation, differentiation, and survival [8].

• Interleukin 8 IL-8, also known as *neutrophil chemotactic factor,* has two functions. It is the GPS for cells to migrate to a needed place (site of infection) and then when they get there it directs them to become packmen and chew up any bad tissue [9][10]

• keratinocyte growth factor. This growth factor is the instructor to give direction for the skin to cover the wound [11].

• connective tissue growth factor (CTGF) This growth factor has many important roles in several biological processes, including cell adhesion (cells sticking to each other), cell movement, recent cell growth, and new blood vessels. All are important in tissue wound repair [12][13][14].

Figure 15: Plasma portion of blood is yellow

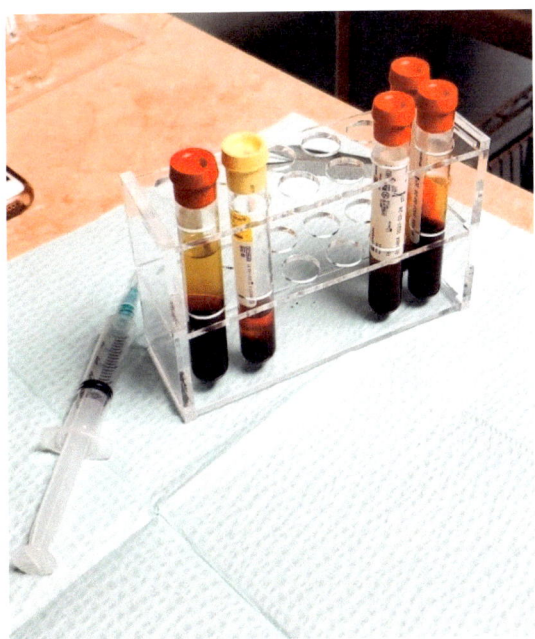

The above list may bore you to tears, but if you scan it, you can see that PRP is full of healing and smart chemicals.

This is the start of what we know about PRP. Only six years ago, there were seven growth factors and now there are 15. The list above is what scientists have been able to identify so far. There is much more to learn about PRP.

Let's go back to when you skin your knee. The first step in this healing process is for the scrape to clot. This process called thrombosis, uses a chemical called thrombin. Thrombin promotes coagulation and causes growth factors to proliferate. It also promotes inflammation. Inflammation helps the cells to stick to the area, and turn on certain cells necessary for healing. Everyone thinks inflammation is bad, but it is necessary for healing. The problem with inflammation is when it becomes chronic and you have a situation where inflammation never resolves itself.

Inflammation is a cascade of chemical reactions. After a series of these chemical reactions, they produce a group of chemicals called prostaglandins. Prostaglandins cause pain.

Check out the diagram.

Diagram 1: Inflammation and healing pathway

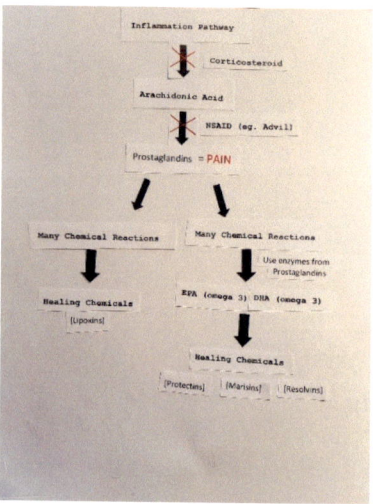

The prostaglandins produced in the middle of the pathway cause pain. A corticosteroid stops pain for a while because it interrupts the series of chemical reactions right at the start of the inflammatory pathway. Non-steroidal anti-inflammatories (e.g. Advil) interrupt the inflammatory pathway too, but further down the pathway. They, too, inhibit the pain causing prostaglandins. The problem is enzymes produced from prostaglandins turn on a healing pathway. These enzymes trigger a complete set of healing chemicals. So, inflammation and healing work in unison. In essence, arresting the inflammatory pathway inactivates the healing pathway. Chemicals called specialized Pro-resolving mediators or as I like to call them Healing Chemicals (resolvins, protectins, marisins and lipoxins) start the healing pathway. A chemical reaction with EPA (Eicosapentanoic Acid) and DHA (Docosahexanoic Acid) your omega 3s, create resolvins and protectins.

EPA and DHA come from cold water fish. The omega 3s everybody talks about are important for your ability to heal. Lipoxins come from a second inflammatory pathway that forks near the beginning of the inflammatory pathway. Researchers discovered the pathway with the use of aspirin. Therefore, much of the literature calls the chemicals aspirin triggered lipoxins (ATL).

The first step with activated PRP is inflammation but then it turns to cell proliferation and tissue regeneration. In other words, healing!

References for Chapter 3:

1.  Hannink, M., & Donoghue, D.J. (1989). Structure and function of platelet-derived growth factor (PDGF) and related proteins. *Biochimica et biophysica acta, 989*(1), 1-10. DOI:10.1016/0304-419x(89)90031-0. PMID 2546599.

2.  Roberts, A.B., Kim, S.J., Noma, T., Glick, A.B., Lafyatis, R., Lechleider, R., ... & Danielpour, D. (1991). Multiple forms of TGF-beta: distinct promoters and differential expression. *Ciba Foundation symposium, 157*,7-15;discussion15-28. DOI:10.1002/9780470514061.ch2. PMID 1906395.

3.  Ornitz, D.M., & Itoh, N. (2001). Fibroblast growth factors. *Genome biology, 2*(3), REVIEWS3005. DOI:10.1186/gb-2001-2-3-reviews3005.

    PMID 11276432.

4.  Reuss, B., & von Bohlen und Halbach, O. (2003). Fibroblast growth factors and their receptors in the central nervous system. *Cell and tissue research, 313*(2), 139-57. DOI:10.1007/s00441-003-0756-7. PMID 12845521.

5.  Yakar, S., Rosen, C.J., Beamer, W.G., Ackert-Bicknell, C.L., Wu, Y., Liu, J.L., ... & LeRoith, D. (2002). Circulating levels of IGF-1 directly regulate bone growth and density. The *Journal of clinical investigation, 110*(6), 771-81. DOI:10.1172/JCI15463. PMID 12235108.

6.  "Insulin-Like Growth Factor II." MeSH. NCBI.

7. Palmer, B.F., & Clegg, D.J. (2014). Oxygen sensing and metabolic homeostasis. *Molecular and cellular endocrinology, 397*(1-2), 51-8. DOI:10.1016/j.mce.2014.08.001. PMID 25132648.

8. Carpenter, G., & Cohen, S. (1990). Epidermal growth factor. *The Journal of biological chemistry, 265*(14), 7709-12. PMID 2186024.

9. Modi, W.S., Dean, M., Seuanez, H.N., Mukaida, N., Matsushima, K., & O'Brien, S.J. (1990). Monocyte-derived neutrophil chemotactic factor (MDNCF/IL-8) resides in a gene cluster along with several other members of the platelet factor 4 gene superfamily. *Human genetics, 84*(2), 185-7. DOI:10.1007/BF00208938. PMID 1967588.

10. "Entrez Gene: IL8 interleukin 8."

11. Rotolo, S., Ceccarelli, S., Romano, F., Frati, L., Marchese, C., & Angeloni, A. (2008). Silencing of keratinocyte growth factor receptor restores 5-fluorouracil and tamoxifen efficacy on responsive cancer cells. *PloS one, 3*(6), e2528. DOI:10.1371/journal.pone.0002528. PMID 18575591.

12. Jun, J.I., & Lau, L.F. (2011). Taking aim at the extracellular matrix: CCN proteins as emerging therapeutic targets. *Nature reviews. Drug discovery, 10*(12), 945-63. DOI:10.1038/nrd3599. PMID 22129992.

13. Hall-Glenn, F., & Lyons, K.M. (2011). Roles for CCN2 in normal physiological processes. *Cellular and molecular life*

*sciences: CMLS, 68*(19), 3209-17. DOI:10.1007/s00018-011-0782-7. PMID 21858450.

14. Kubota, S., & Takigawa, M. (2011). The role of CCN2 in cartilage and bone development. *Journal of cell communication and signaling, 5*(3), 209-17. DOI:10.1007/s12079-011-0123-5. PMID 21484188.

# CHAPTER 4:
# VAMPIRE FACELIFT® AND VAMPIRE FACIAL®

The Vampire procedures use all the scientific principles you've read so far. Healing occurs the same way it would be if you skin your knee. Vampire Facial® uses the same PRP that your body uses naturally to heal. It places the concentrated healing factors in your face and your skin heals. New blood vessels improve the color and tone of the skin. New collagen gives more structure under the skin. As we age, our skin falls and gets closer to the bone. The collagen picks up the skin and gives it better structure. PRP decreases pore size and fine lines disappear. Beauty fads come and go, but this is a healing procedure. All the things PRP does when you skin your knee is what it does for your face.

Let's look at two growth factors:

Platelet-derived growth factor triggers cell growth and cell division. What that means for your facial skin is new skin, which makes you younger in an instant. Many of us do not recognize how sallow and gray we have become because it is a gradual change. We lose the luster and rosy coloring in our skin and don't even recognize it. PRP plays a substantial role in the blood vessel formation. The grayness that creeps up on our skin over time is reversed. Fresh blood flow helps to rejuvenate the skin's coloring. The skin has a youthful glow that is almost indescribable.

This is a scientific beauty treatment.

There are so many growth factors it is difficult to isolate one versus another. But let's look at one more growth factor transforming growth factor beta (TGF-beta). It has a crucial role in attracting stem cells and directing them to become what we need. This is a critical growth factor. It helps to form new cells in the epidermis, dermis, blood vessels, and collagen. Any new cell needed to repair damage and restore health involves this growth factor, TGF beta.

In three treatments or fewer, you will have smaller pore size, less dry skin, fewer wrinkles, thicker under eye skin, plumper overall skin and more.

It is much more than this, though. I joke with my husband, "Where did all the color go?" My hair is no longer brown, my eyebrows are disappearing and both are turning gray. My skin was also turning gray, but I did not see it until I healed my skin with PRP. People now remark how good my skin looks and only one thing has changed–three Vampire Facial(s) ®.

There are many growth factors that work to enhance and stimulate repair and rejuvenation.

Some words that come to mind after a Vampire Facial ® are glow, radiant, radiance, luminosity, brilliance, shine, sparkle, happiness, vivacity, warmth, enthusiasm, oomph, gleam, polish, and luster!

**Dermal Fillers vs Botox**

Let's talk about dermal fillers vs Botox. Many women I talk to fear dermal fillers because they see the odd faces of Hollywood. There is an artistic way to use dermal filler and a non-artistic way. Here's why.

Beauty is mathematical. Yes, you read that right, it IS mathematical.

Early in my dental career, I learned about the golden proportion. The Golden Proportion is 1 to 1.618. Let me explain. The correct proportion of the front tooth to the lateral tooth (the second tooth) is 1.618 to 1. The front tooth being 1.618 and the 2nd tooth is 1. It doesn't stop with the front two teeth. The second tooth is in that exact ratio to the third tooth. Here is a picture of a gauge to measure the correct proportion of the two front teeth described above.

Figure 16: Golden proportion dental ruler

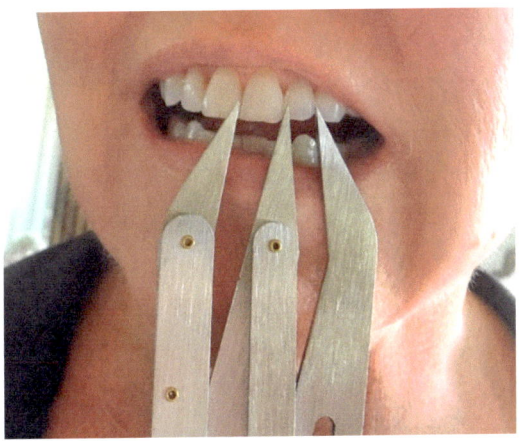

But we find the golden proportion throughout nature. We find it in snail shells, flowers, faces, and more.

Figure 17: Golden Proportion in nature

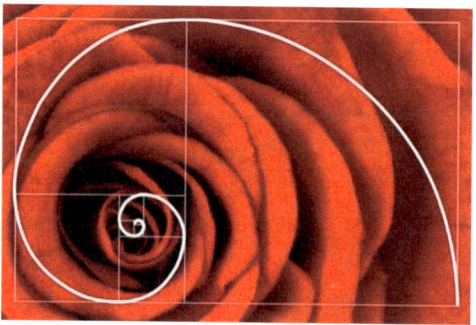

A guy named Marquardt drew a mask of the golden rule, otherwise known as the golden proportion of the human face. It has stood the test of time for beauty. It does not matter if it is antiquity or modern day, the human brain finds the same proportions beautiful. You can Google this subject and find a lot of evidence for mathematical beauty. But if someone distorts these proportions, you can spot it instantly. When I see someone with overfilled dermal filler, I almost have a jerking reaction. It is disturbing. Some people do not want any wrinkles. The face becomes distorted to remove all wrinkles.

Hyaluronic acid or calcium hydroxyapatite which are both found naturally in the human body, composes dermal filler. The products have varying thicknesses for different uses and areas of the face. To inject the dermal filler, the provider needs training and must have a good artistic eye. There is no need to OVER fill the cheeks, the lips or any other part of the face.

My advice is to go to someone with an artistic eye that sees the whole face. And do not OVER fill! Less is more.

Pictures help to explain the aging changes that dermal filler can correct.

Figure 18: Dermal Filler helps to smooth skin by supporting it.

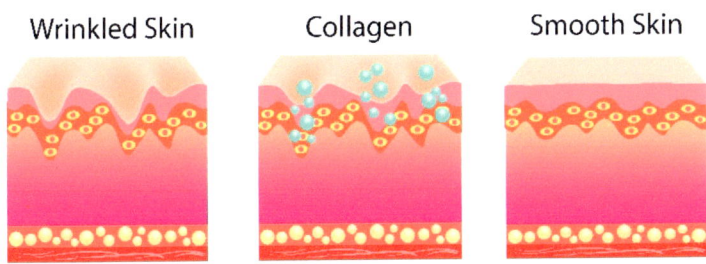

Wrinkled Skin      Collagen      Smooth Skin

There is a break that occurs under our eyes as we age. This line makes us look tired and older. Filling cheeks can have a significant impact on how tired we look. It also affects the lower third of the face by lifting it at the same time. We can decrease the sad line, as I like to call it. Here is an excellent example of what dermal filler can do to enhance the face not distort it.

Figure 19: Before and After Dermal Filler, Botox and Vampire Facial

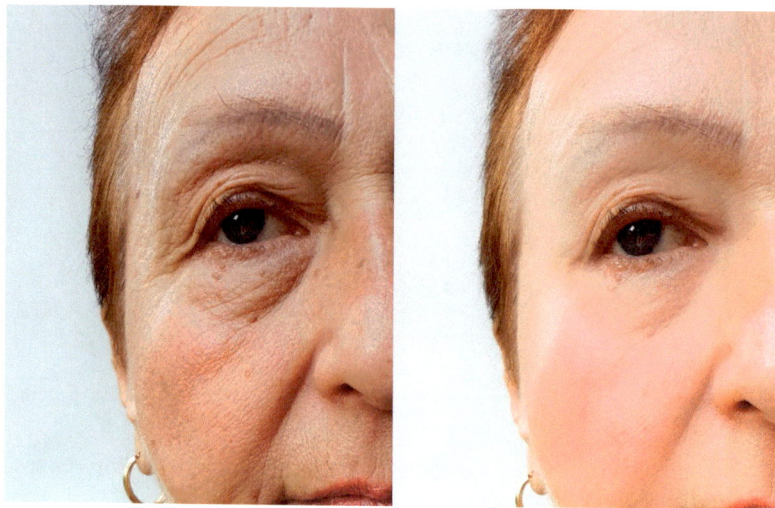

The "marionette" line or puppet mouth, starts at the corner of the mouth and follows to the jaw line. This also contributes to a sad look. This is a splendid place to use dermal filler. Here is an example:

Figure 20: Before and After a series of Dermal Filler appointments

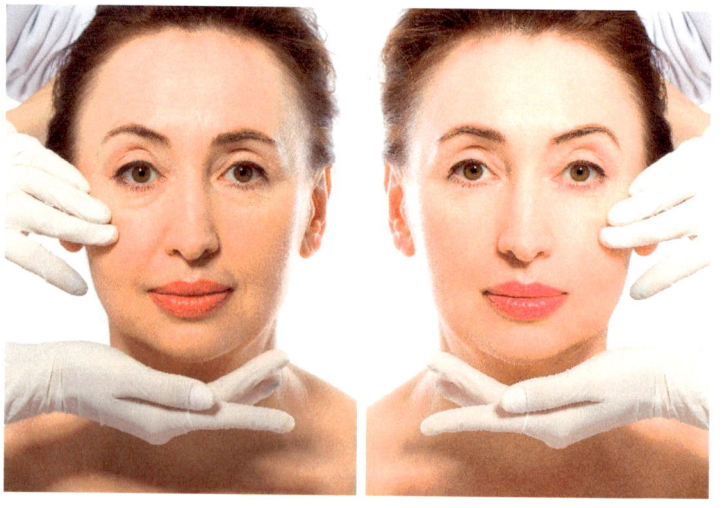

An interesting area that has more impact on the face than you would think is sunken temples. Not everyone gets this aging feature but sunken in temples scream old age, and when filled in, they brighten and add youthfulness.

Let's talk about lips. There has been a trend in the fashion industry that bigger is better. Not so. Lips have a natural shape. They go in and out throughout the upper and lower lip. The trend toward making the lips two big sausages is unfortunate. The brain immediately recognizes the misshapen lips. This diagram will help explain what I mean

Diagram 2: Lips have a natural flow no matter the size

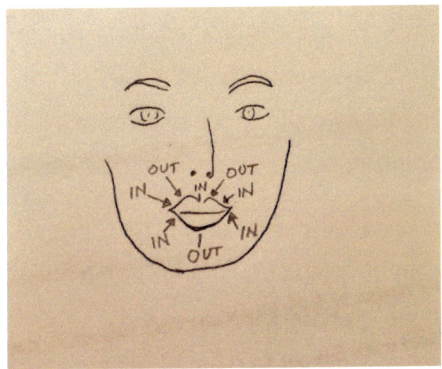

There is also a natural profile for lips. The upper lip should not be bigger than the lower lip. When it is, you know it. You may not know what is wrong, but you know something does not look right.

This drawing shows the correct profile relationship and an incorrect profile relationship.

Diagram 3: Natural profile, the upper lip is smaller than the lower lip

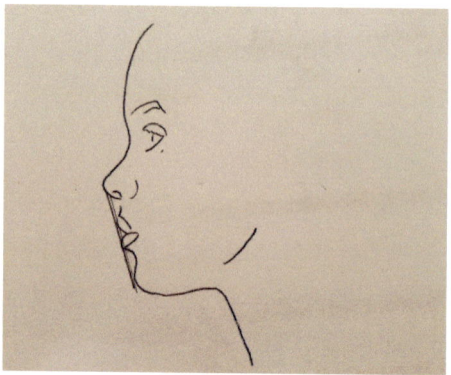

A natural way to enhance lips is to recreate the border with filler. As we age, the border of the lips gets fuzzy and less defined. It is a subtle but substantive enhancement. These may seem like little and unimportant changes but combined they make all the difference in you looking rested and more vibrant.

The human condition suggests that we are more likely to "buy" from who is vibrant and attractive. I didn't say beautiful. I said vibrant and attractive. It may not be fair, but we are hard-wired in certain decision-making ways. This is subconscious and driven by genetics. Taking care of your vibrancy and attractiveness will help you in any business. If you do not think you are a salesperson in life, think again. In every job, you sell someone on something. A manager sells the alternative system she wants her employees to use. A mom sells a million little things and ideas all day long to her children. The more you take care of yourself the more people listen and agree with you.

Dermal filler is used to add volume, for example, cheeks, nasolabial area, marionette lines, and lips.

So, when you combine dermal filler and PRP, it is the best of all worlds. Dermal filler helps the sagging volume, and the PRP rejuvenates the skin.

## Botox

Botox is a neurotoxin that paralyses the muscles. As you contract muscles you pull the skin together. After enough time, the skin does not have the elasticity to bounce back, and it shows where the skin was pulled together with wrinkles. If we stop the muscles from contracting, we stop pulling on the skin and the skin smooths back out. The difference between dermal filler and Botox is dermal filler increases the volume under the skin and Botox freezes muscles to keep the skin from being pulled together. To correct the 11's or horizontal wrinkles, we primarily use Botox on the forehead.

When you see someone, whose face appears stuck and mask-like, they have used too much Botox all over the face. People with crow's feet and the fine lip wrinkles may enjoy Botox but it takes precision not to overdo it. You want to move in a natural manner. Everything has its place and possible enhancement, but there are limits. Many people push the limits and fall off the beauty cliff.

Some people think the forehead is important for facial expression and it is not. The eyes are the most important source of expression, which is why we call them the window to the soul.

There are some recent uses for Botox. It is being used for migraines and tension headaches. It works well for many people. People who receive Botox for migraines report they stopped getting headaches when they started getting Botox. I have found that most tension headache sufferers receiving Botox on the forehead alone rids them of their headaches. Twenty percent of patients need Botox added to the back of the skull to relieve them of tension headaches.

The hard part about Botox is that it lasts for 3-4 months and those with headaches know when it is wearing off. The maintenance is a lot more than dermal fillers that last anywhere from 12 months to two years.

# CHAPTER 5:
# RESEARCH AT OUR FINGERTIPS

I have scoured Pubmed.com (National Library of Medicine National Institute of Health) for every study I can find where the researchers use PRP to treat anything.

The medical community uses PRP in dental bone grafts, orthopedic sports medicine and equine medicine. I joke that if you want the best medicine follow horse medicine. They get the best medicine. (We base all funny things on truth.)

My husband and I live on four acres and our neighbor has three horses which are gorgeous, but a ton of work. We only have four chickens and one dog. When I mentioned to the neighbor that I was using PRP for a Vampire Facial®, she said, "Oh, yeah for the last 15 years the vet suggests PRP anytime they think a horse has hurt their leg tendon or ligament."

Most people I talk to have never heard of PRP unless they have had a sports injury and the surgeon has offered PRP for the surgical site. Anytime the horses hurt, they receive restorative injections! We should do the same. Could we reduce the amount of arthritis? Reduce aches and pains? Reduce immobility because of injury?

There are many studies on the uses of PRP in various applications going back to the early 1990s for dental bone grafts. Studies show up for skin uses around 2004. Researchers started looking at hair restoration in 2010. As far as a medical treatment, it is new in a historical sense. The other obstacle that has slowed down its use is that medical insurance won't pay for it.

I don't want to get on my soapbox but allow me one comment. If medical insurance ever gets in the mix and pays for it, the price will skyrocket. Period. My costs to verify insurance and find out what dental insurance pays for and what they don't are more than I pay for one employee a day in the dental office. It drives my dental fees up. That is a fact.

What I love about PRP, is that it is your healing factors being concentrated in an area that needs healing. It is one of the safest medical procedures, but recognize it is in infancy.

There was a news report from a "medspa" in New Mexico where two customers contracted AIDS from a Vampire Facial®. What? Cannot happen with good sterile procedures and proper equipment. My wonderful friend sent me a photo of that Medspa. It tells the entire story-VIP SPA. Look at the "I."Figure 21: Front door of the VIP Spa

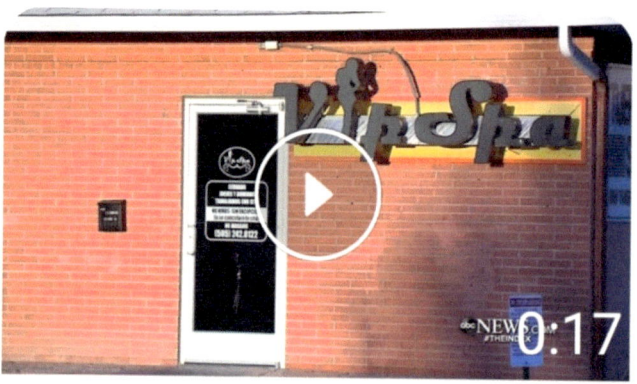

Say no more!

The Vampire Facial® uses your Platelet Rich Plasma from your own blood and we inject it into your face. Many aestheticians may not have a license to inject. If they cannot inject, they smear PRP on the outside and use the skin-pen to introduce it into the skin. The skin-pen is a medical device that contains needles to pierce the skin and cause microtrauma.

Microtrauma is another way to induce the body to start the healing process. You cause a little trauma to induce the healing cascade. There are several ways to introduce a slight amount of trauma, including the skin-pen, a laser, or radiofrequency (heat) to name a few.

Just know some providers call the micro-needling and putting PRP on the skin surface a Vampire Facial® but it is not, and it is minimally effective. Micro-needling plus *injecting* PRP is the real deal. This is not an over promising beauty product. It delivers.

This natural healing process concentrates in the face where it heals your skin. The best part is the procedure's safety. We inject no foreign substances. It is YOU HEALING YOU! When advertisers claim all natural, organic, local, this truly is natural, organic, and local. The fountain of youth is right inside of you.

And damn, the skin looks wonderful.

**Facial Cream**

I found a study where they looked at PRP infused cream on lip wrinkles and thought it was very interesting, but there are some difficulties making a cream out of your PRP.[1] First, there are studies that show PRP is stable for about one week, even at room temperature. Well, think about it--PRP normal temperature is 98.6 degrees–body temperature. Did studied participants give blood every week to make the cream? Seems unlikely.

With a little more investigation, we discover frozen PRP is stable. [2] That's how they did it. The researchers froze PRP for six months. They thawed it and tested to see if it were the same. It stayed consistent with all those glorious healing factors, proteins and hormones for six months. That is how we can make a cream and the eye drops. More about eye drops later in the book.

We make a cream with PRP and freeze it. You use it for one week. At the end of the week you take another aliquot of cream out of the freezer.

I have seen my major lip wrinkle soften after about 12–15 weeks. This is exciting.

Isn't it great you get to put your natural healing factors on your skin to give it a chance to heal naturally the way God meant it to?

Let's look at some other conditions that used PRP as the "medicine." This compilation will give you the knowledge of an alternative treatment. These conditions have one trait in common: there aren't excellent treatments available in medical practice today for each of them. The reason for this book is to inform you of one excellent and safe alternative treatment that may or may not help. It is important that people know about PRP as a viable alternative.

References for Chapter 5:

1. Draelos, Z.D., Rheins, L.A., Wootten, S., Kellar, R.S., & Diller, R.B.(in press). Pilot study: Autologous platelet-rich plasma used in a topical cream for facial rejuvenation. *Journal of cosmetic dermatology.* DOI:10.1111/jocd.13088

2. Kaux, J.F., Libertiaux, V., Dupont, L., Colige, A., Denoël, V., Lecut, C., ... & Drion, P. (2020). Platelet-rich plasma (PRP) and tendon healing: comparison between fresh and frozen-thawed PRP. *Platelets,* 31(2), 221-5. PMID: 30915890

   DOI: 10.1080/09537104.2019.1595563

# CHAPTER 6:
# BEYOND ESTHETICS-MEDICAL USES FOR PRP

The next part of this book explores other uses for PRP. It examines case studies and investigates published research. There are many conditions that have no or poor treatments and less than desirable treatment outcomes. What if there is a treatment right inside of all of us? One clinical observation that needs mentioning is that when we treat a recent injury with PRP, the response is intense and immediate. The long-term injuries seem to take multiple PRP sessions but there are some significant results.

**Bell's Palsy**

Now that we have seen a scar all but disappear and a tendon that repaired itself, what else can PRP heal?

I was talking to my dental supply representative. He came over to see my extra space and check it out. I explained to him about the Vampire Facial® and told him all the remarkable things we have observed. I had a dental patient with Bell's Palsy that I had talked to about trying PRP for the residual symptoms. She was a little chicken to get injections, so I had not convinced her to try it. I don't know why I brought it up, but I told him I wanted to do a study on Bell's Palsy. He said, "I have Bell's Palsy." The universe was at work again.

A study was published in 2017 where one patient with Bell's Palsy received PRP treatment with noted improvement [1]. This patient developed Bell's Palsy as a six-months-old baby. The PRP treatment started when she was 27 years old. Because she had Bell's Palsy at such a young age, the palsy affected her facial growth pattern.

The researchers injected a little over 1 cc to each injection site. They distributed PRP to the right side of the face following the pattern of the 7th cranial nerve. They repeated these injections nine times within one year. There was significant improvement in voluntary movement with the facial muscles and there was a reduction in asymmetry on the right and left sides of the face. One of the most remarkable improvements was her new ability to close her left eyelid and close her right eye over 80%.

Figure 22: Before and after PRP treatment

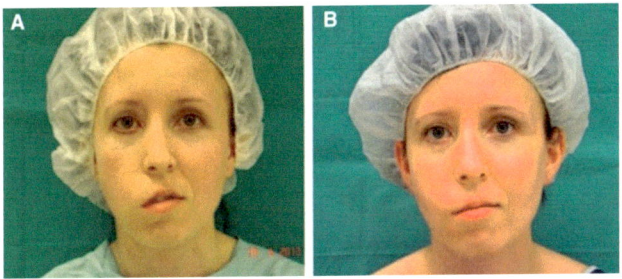

A.      Is before treatment.

B.      Is post treatment–she has more symmetry comparing right and left sides. There is less atrophy on the right side, mostly, the cheek. The corner of her lip rose, too.

Figure 23: Before and after PRP treatment

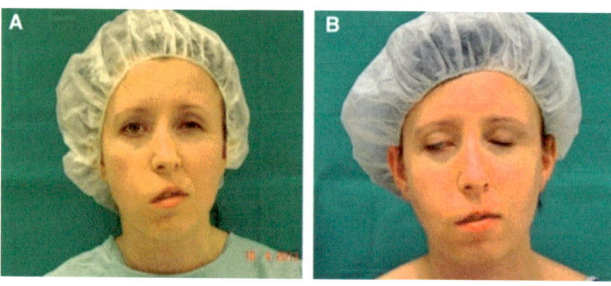

A.      Patient closing eyes before treatment.

B.      Patient closing left eye 100% and right eye 80%.

Figure 24: Before and After Measurement of the eye closure

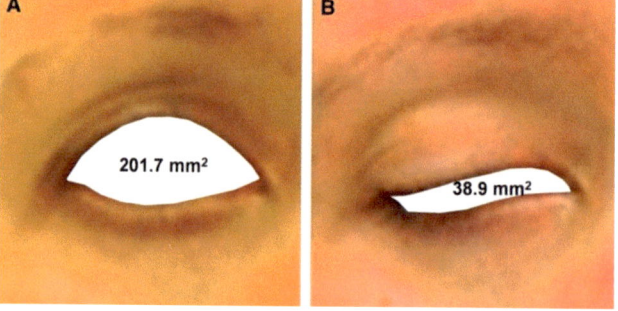

A.      Measurement of eye closure before treatment.

B.      Measurement of eye closure after treatment.

The physical facial changes and voluntary muscle movement improvements are remarkable in this case, considering the patient had the residual effects of Bell's palsy for so many years.

It had never crossed my mind that my dental rep had Bell's Palsy. I just thought he was a Texan that talked out of the side of his mouth. He explained to me that he has had residual effects from Bell's Palsy for

27 years. One of the worst residual symptoms was tremendous light sensitivity. He could not go outside without sunglasses. I threw him into the treatment chair to inject PRP into the affected side. I'm kidding. He wanted to at least try to see if it made any difference.

Bell's Palsy is paralysis of the 7th cranial nerve. If you place the heel of your hand by your ear with your thumb up and your pointer finger on your eyebrow and fan your fingers down the face evenly you are following the course of the 7th cranial nerve. Skull with 7th cranial nerve in red.

Diagram 4: 7th Cranial nerve

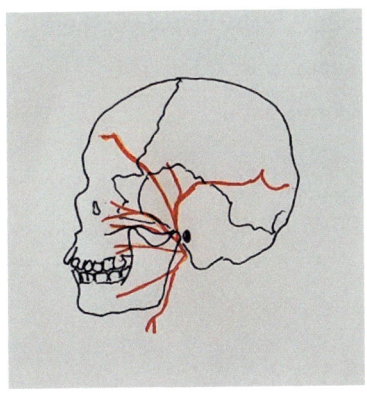

I injected PRP where the 7th cranial nerve runs similar to the study cited above. I have watched PRP go to where it needs to go. Just get it in the general area and it goes where it needs to go to repair what it needs to repair. I have submitted this case to the Annals of Case Reports to spread this information into the scientific community.

Within one week, the dental rep reported he was less sensitive to light. He could walk outside without sunglasses , which he had not done in 27 years. What a life-changing improvement. His eye became more open and not as droopy. He loves it. Among his positive remarks, he stated he had more peripheral vision. The dental rep hadn't realized how much peripheral vision he lost until he got it back. His lip movement also improved, and he reported better articulation.

One odd symptom that most do not know about Bell's Palsy is that the eye on the affected side will tear when the person eats. This is one of the most frustrating symptoms for the patient. After the second treatment, he stopped tearing when he ate.

We treated him twice, and he improved with every treatment. Remember this is 27 years after someone diagnosed him first with Bell's palsy, and it had not changed since his initial recovery period.

Most patients recover from the original Bell's Palsy attack but there are over 15 - 20% that have remaining symptoms. This is a life changing treatment the world needs to know about.

I contacted Dr. Seffer, the researcher in the study of the young woman, to ask if I could publish his pictures. He was kind enough to share some other successful cases.

Figure 25: Bell's Palsy treated with PRP

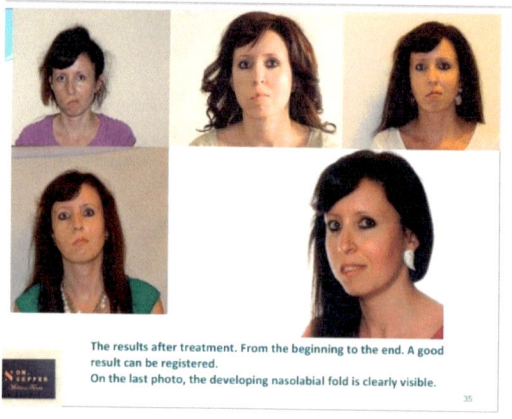

The results after treatment. From the beginning to the end. A good result can be registered.
On the last photo, the developing nasolabial fold is clearly visible.

Figure: 26: Bell's Palsy patient treated with PRP

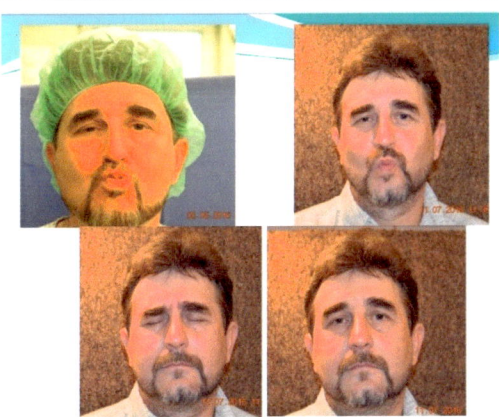

Case No. 3: 54 yrs old male patient, who was suffering from a minor left side Bell
condition started at age of 54 years. After a thorough medical investigation (checl
symplex was suspected as cause of infection. Usual treatments have not resulted ii
After a month, autologue PBMC plasma treatment was used. He reported a dram
in 5 days.

References for Chapter 6:

1. Seffer, I., & Nemeth, Z. (2017). Recovery from Bell Palsy after Transplantation of Peripheral Blood Mononuclear Cells and Platelet-Rich Plasma. *Plastic and reconstructive surgery. Global open,* 5(6), e1376.

# CHAPTER 7:
# MUSCLE PAIN

A friend of mine has some serious degeneration of his spine. He beat the crap out of his body as a strong youthful man and now his body is telling him so. His first job at 17 years old was a bricklayer. Because he is tall, his job was to hold the bricks in a tower with a straight arm above his head to deliver the bricks to the bricklayers. That repetitive movement hurt his shoulders. He also was a serious snow skier, and a competitive windsurfer. The activities took a toll on his body and his back. He has been in constant back pain for most of his adult life.

The MRI told the story with one word: degeneration. Throughout the report of each area studied, the analysis suggested severe degeneration.

This friend underwent a PRP treatment a few years ago when he flew in from Houston to Florida. It was successful, and he was symptom free for a few years.

His treatment for pain consisted of nerve blocks. The blocks lasted for a little while, but the pain always returned. He also tried Radiofrequency ablation (RFA) on the nerve pain. An electrical current produced by a radio wave is used to heat a small area of nerve tissue decreasing the nerve signals sent to the brain, decreasing pain. But this procedure did not last. He scheduled another RFA procedure but changed his mind and asked us to inject his spine muscles with PRP. After the healing I have seen, I agreed we could inject next to his spine in the muscle with PRP, not into the joints of the spine.

I found a very interesting pilot study that injected PRP into the masseter muscle (facial muscle) to see if it would reduce facial pain for TMJ (Temporomandibular Joint [Disorder]) patients. [1] TMJ is a condition where the jaw joint may click or pop; however, the patient experiences an excessive amount of head and neck pain. The study showed significant results. Almost 60% of the PRP group reduced muscle pain within five days as opposed to the control group which received an injection of saline only. They only had about 10% reduction of pain. PRP helped facial muscles. Why wouldn't back muscles respond the same way?

He came in and we injected next to his spine all the way down about an inch from the spine into muscles. Within 1 week, he reported feeling much better. He says he can relax his back muscles for the first time in a long time. The muscles responded just as the facial muscles did in the study cited above. He reported he could tolerate much more in life.

Three weeks after the treatment he had to drive to Midland from Houston. Texas is a big state. It is only an eight-hour drive. Lol. He was excited to tell me that the drive was okay. He says he could not have done that before the injections without being in severe pain for days after the drive. Three days later it was eight hours back home. This would be rough on anyone but he did it without being out of commission, in bed and in severe pain, for days following the trip.

He had already reported that his pelvis always shifted out of alignment and he must get chiropractic adjustments to realign it. Since the first treatment on his spinal muscles, his pelvis has stayed in alignment. An interesting observation.

Feeling better, he wanted to inject the muscles of his shoulders, in and around both shoulders. He came in six weeks after the first treatment on his back to inject his shoulders. The shoulders did not get better. PRP has been fantastic, but it has limitations. The most important part is to have a good diagnosis. Is the damaged tendon-related, ligament-related, bone damage, joint space inadequacies or something else? There are other tools in a practitioner's hands. For example, hyaluronic acid (the same thing used as dermal filler) increases fluid in the joint space. Stem cells is another possibility when looking to rebuild an area of the body.

References for Chapter 7:

1. Nitecka-Buchta, A., Walczynska-Dragon, K., Kempa, W.M., & Baron, S. (2019). Platelet-Rich Plasma Intramuscular Injections - Antinociceptive Therapy in Myofascial Pain Within Masseter Muscles in Temporomandibular Disorders Patients: A Pilot Study. *Frontiers in neurology,* 10, 250. PMID 30941095

# CHAPTER 8:
# THE TOE NAIL

Nobody gets away without seeing my toenail. As you know, I retired from practicing dentistry, but I am still involved in running the dental practice. The entire dental staff (there are 20) all say, "Yes, Dr. Cody I have seen your toenail." It is such a great visual of the healing capabilities of PRP.

This has been two years of the big toenails. Last year at a great yoga studio called Yoga on the Brazos, I was on all fours, rolling up my yoga mat, and I slid my right leg along the floor and ripped my big toenail off. There was an odd piece of molding attached to the floor that covered patched flood damage. The injury stunned me, and I did not even make a sound. I limped out and drove home with blood dripping from the injury. It took a full year for the toenail to grow back. No pedicures for me.

The next year, we went on a family snow skiing trip. My left boot was too tight. I have snow skied my entire life. There isn't any excuse. I was being lazy. My toe hurt when I skied, but I still did not change my boots. No. I kept skiing. If you have never skied, you cannot just change boots. You must have the ski bindings readjusted. It wasn't an enormous deal, but I just kept skiing.

Within a week of being home, my toenail turned black. Oh no, I will lose another toenail. Well, I lost half of it. I trimmed the part of the nail that was no longer attached to the nail bed and left the part that was stuck. Over the years, I have met several women who leave the part of the nail that is off the nail bed and paint the nail to hide it.

Knowing me, I would catch the toenail on something and rip it off. I lived that pain and nightmare the year before.

One day Glenna and I started experimenting with PRP. I said to her, "Why don't we put it in my toe and see if we can heal my big toenail faster?"

The first photo is of my toenail four 1/2 months after the ski trip. It had grown about 4 mm. This would be a long year of no flip flops.

*Add note: The growth of the nail in 4 months. The bruised area was the nail attached to the bed. The area with no nail—I trimmed off.*

Figure 27: My big toe before treatment with PRP

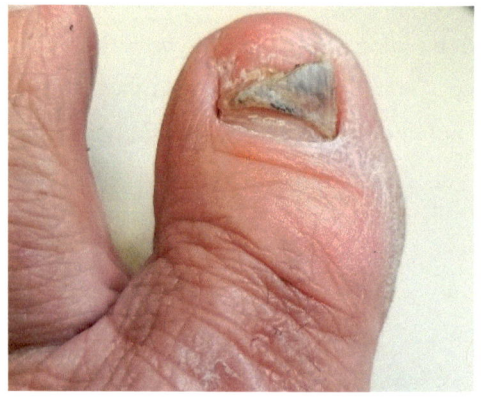

I try to go to yoga three to four times a week. I am barefoot a bunch and I live in Houston. We wear flip flops most of the time. I thought I would have to wear closed toe shoes for a year or more.

I was in yoga about three weeks after the PRP injection and I almost fainted. The black part of the bruise disappeared. The toenail looked much better.

Figure 28: 3 weeks after PRP treatment

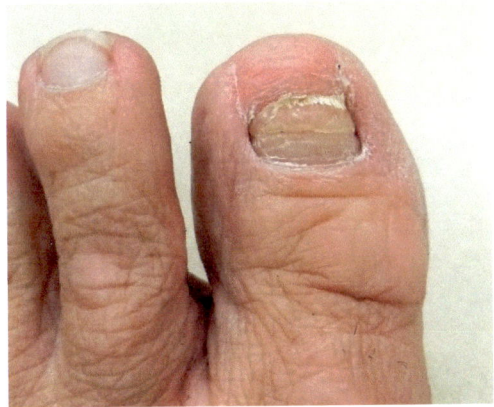

Before PRP and three weeks after 1 PRP treatment.

I have never bruised a nail and did not have to cut off the bruised areas as it grew out. The nail healed in an instant.

Have you ever seen a nail heal at that rate? Neither have I. I love that it is such a visual of the power of what PRP does.

It is hard to see how much better a bone graft has integrated. One just knows it is ready for a dental implant, and the x-ray shows bone in the extraction area but you cannot see the healing.

It is hard to know that when the doctor uses PRP in an orthopedic surgery, it helps in healing. But we can all see a toenail!

Before, three weeks and six weeks after PRP treatment. Even my skin looks better.

Figure :29: Before, 3 weeks after PRP treatment and 6 weeks after PRP treatment

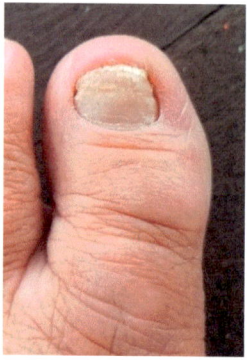

I could get a pedicure within 10 weeks of PRP treatment.

I knew there would not be any study on toenails but for grins I searched and voila! Researchers published one in March 2019. The researchers injected PRP into the matrix of the toenail on two patients with nail disorders. One patient had lichen striatus and the other patient had idiopathic trachyonychia. Both disorders look like ridged, peeling nails. The researchers injected 1.0 cc of PRP three times one week apart. And then they followed up at 16 and 20 weeks. Both patients saw improvement. One saw improvement within three weeks and the other in six weeks. Neither patient relapsed at 20 weeks.

I observed at 12 weeks that my nail didn't grow as fast. That was another interesting observation.

# CHAPTER 9:
# HAIR

H air regrowth is another improvement. Many practitioners are aware of treating hair loss either from male pattern balding or female hair loss with PRP. It takes multiple treatments, usually, three treatments four to six weeks apart with maintenance treatments every six to twelve months.

I had a patient with alopecia areata which is an autoimmune disorder that causes hair loss most often on the scalp and beard but can occur on any part of the body. He had lost a swath of hair on his head and it looked like a reverse Mohawk. He is only 14 years old, so his mother wanted to get some hair growth back. The picture shows how many new hairs were visible in five weeks.

Figure 30: Before Treatment / 5 weeks post treatment.

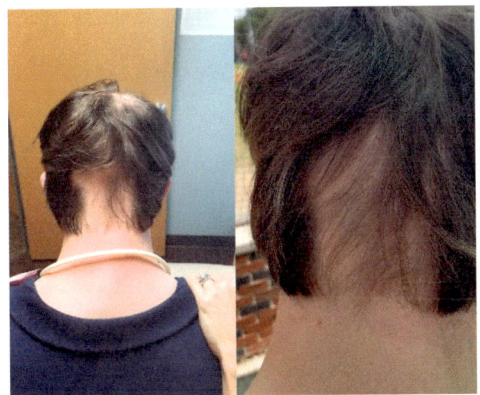

The earliest study using PRP as a treatment for alopecia areata was 2013. The bulk of published studies took place in the last couple of years. This means a very new treatment for this immune disorder.

PRP treatment is an excellent non-surgical, low risk treatment that has an excellent track record for other causes of baldness and worth trying.

Female pattern baldness responds very well to PRP treatment.

Funny Story- I have had psoriasis since the day I was born. If you know anything about psoriasis, you know it comes and goes. But last summer it came with a vengeance. Psoriatic plaques covered my scalp. They itched constantly and incessantly, nonstop. This was the worst it had been in years. Desperate for relief I had my nurse, Glenna, inject my entire head with Platelet Rich Plasma (PRP). It was worth a try.

Over the next 12 weeks, the psoriatic plaques disappeared one by one, and the itching decreased daily. This was marvelous news. I have only found one research paper on psoriasis and PRP, but I wanted to try it.

I know you are saying, "Where is the funny part?" Well, here it is... I was pulling my hair back in a ponytail and noticed all these hairs sticking up all over my head. I kept trying to smooth them down and they would pop back up. Weird! Then I realized I had new hair growth from the PRP. Here are a couple of pictures:

Figure 31: New hair growth after PRP

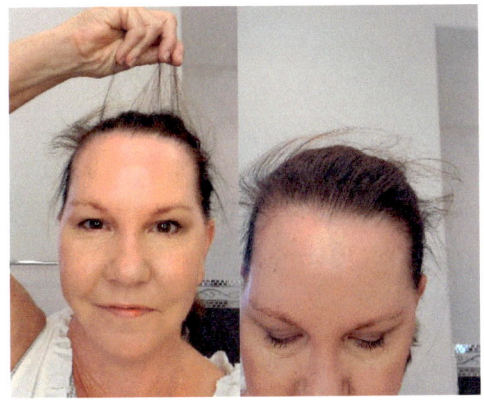

The first hair that grows is fine baby hairs and then they mature.

# CHAPTER 10:
# DRY EYES

I did not realize until I consulted with the optometrist how serious dry eyes can be. It is a serious problem, for example, for those diagnosed with Sjogren syndrome. The long-term effects can cause permanent eye damage so a treatment could be valuable.

There are studies using PRP as eyedrops. The eyedrops are not diluted. It is straight PRP. The studies for eyes call them PRGF, Plasma Rich Growth Factors, which is more correct than using the term PRP.

Practitioners keep PRP eyedrops fresh by freezing the drops until they are ready for use. One 12-week protocol for dry eyes uses PRP or PRGF eyedrops in a stepwise fashion. The protocol is to use six drops/day of PRP the first week and then reduce to five drops/day the next week to four drops/day, then three drops/day until you stabilize at two drops/day.

After 12 weeks of use, many patients remain symptom free for years and can stop using PRP daily.

You may not need PRP every day, but I can tell you the drops feel like velvet in your eyes. They are soothing and soft (and it can't hurt to allow the PRP to drip on that delicate skin under your eyes–increase collagen, thicken skin, and reduce bags).

I had a patient report after her Vampire Facelift that her eyes were no longer dry. Injecting in the region around the eye helped dry eyes (and reduced wrinkles). A win-win!

A study that followed 26 patients with Sjogren syndrome, an autoimmune disease that causes extreme eye dryness, and other areas, including the mouth, concluded that the patients had significant improvement using PRP. They also stated it was a safe and effective treatment [1]

One of our patients diagnosed with Sjogren reports her ophthalmologist can see the improvement in her eye condition and wants her to continue using PRP. She thinks she has increased visual acuity. "I can see better, especially at night," she said.

Another study compared PRP to artificial tears sodium hyaluronate (SH). The results were outstanding for PRP [2]

Testimonial from patient:

*"I have had dry eyes for a long time. I had to carry vials of eyedrops everywhere and put drops in my eyes all day long. I tried Restasis but did not notice much improvement and it was expensive. In the beginning, I used PRP drops multiple times per day. After 6 weeks, I noticed my right eye feels normal and my left eye is still a little dry but less than it was. The biggest plus is that I now only need 1 drop a day and don't need drops the rest of the day."*

*Angie H.*

A study published in 2018 tested the efficiency of PRP to treat corneal ulcers (neurotropic keratopathy).[3] The study group consisted of 25 patients with non-healing corneal ulcers because of herpes simplex or herpes zoster infection. They instructed the patients to use PRP eyedrops five times per day for three months plus using preservative-free artificial tears and a vitamin A ointment used at night. The researchers looked at four parameters:

1) Best corrected visual acuity (BCVA)
2) Healing of the corneal surface
3) Subjective symptoms
4) Corneal thickness

All patients had improved visual acuity, and all patients reported fewer symptoms. 80% (20 patients) had complete healing of the eye ulcerations. Four patients experienced considerable improvement in reducing the size of the ulceration. One patient experienced no improvement. All the patients' corneal thinning stopped. None of the patients reported general or local side effects of the treatment .

This is remarkable. PRP helped all but one patient to heal NON-HEALING eye ulcers in 12 weeks with no side effects. Realize that all these patients had a condition that was NON-HEALING!

My husband and I both have high intraocular pressure (IOP) and so we were interested in natural ways of bringing down eye pressure. There were two studies by one group of researchers looking at similar parameters as the study mentioned above, however they also measured intraocular pressure. They found that IOP (intraocular pressure) decreased by over 16% over the course of the treatment. The treatment study lasted 22 weeks. At 14 weeks, the corneal ulcers healed in all 6 patients [4].

The fountain of youth or at least the fountain of healing is inside all of us. The eyes are an example of a new area to use PRP. If you or a family member develop non-healing eye ulcers or even dry eye syndrome, here is another avenue to pursue.

References for Chapter 10:

2. Sanchez-Avila, R.M., Merayo-Lloves, J., Riestra, A.C., Anitua, E., Muruzabal, F., Orive, G., & Fernández-Vega, L. (2017). The Effect of Immunologically Safe Plasma Rich in Growth Factor Eye Drops in Patients with Sjögren Syndrome. *Journal of ocular pharmacology and therapeutics : the official journal of the Association for Ocular Pharmacology and Therapeutics,* 33(5), 391-9. PMID:28375790

3. Avila, M.Y., Igua, A.M., & Mora, A.M.(in press). Randomised, prospective clinical trial of platelet-rich plasma injection in the management of severe dry eye. The British journal of *ophthalmology.* DOI:10.1136/bjophthalmol-2018-312072 PMID:29970389

4. Wróbel-Dudzińska, D., Alio, J., Rodriguez, A., Suchodoła-Ratajewicz, E., Kosior-Jarecka, E., Rymgayłło-Jankowska, B., ... & Żarnowski, T. (2018). Clinical Efficacy of Platelet-Rich Plasma in the Treatment of Neurotrophic Corneal Ulcer. *Journal of ophthalmology,* 2018, 3538764. DOI: 10.1155/2018/3538764. eCollection 2018. PMID: 30026985

5. Sánchez-Avila, R.M., Merayo-Lloves, J., Fernández, M.L., Rodríguez-Gutiérrez, L.A., Rodríguez-Calvo, P.P., Fernández-Vega Cueto, A., ... & Anitua, E. (2018). Plasma rich in growth factors eye drops to treat secondary ocular surface disorders in patients with glaucoma. *International medical case reports journal,* 11, 97-103. DOI: 10.2147/IMCRJ.S153918. eCollection 2018PMID: 29760570

6. Miłek, T., Baranowski, K., Zydlewski, P., Ciostek, P., Mlosek, K., & Olszewski, W. (2017). Role of plasma growth factor in the healing of chronic ulcers of the lower legs and foot due to ischaemia in diabetic patients. *Postepy dermatologii i alergologii,* 34(6), 601-6. PMID: 29422826 PMCID: PMC5799748 DOI: 10.5114/pdia.2016.62415

7.  de Leon, J.M., Driver, V.R., Fylling, C.P., Carter, M.J., Anderson, C., Wilson, J., ... & Rappl, L.M. (2011). The Clinical Relevance of Treating Chronic Wounds with an Enhanced Near-Physiological Concentration of Platelet-Rich Plasma Gel. *Advances in Skin & Wound Care*, 24(8), 357-68. DOI: 10.1097/01.ASW.0000403249.85131.6f

8.  Del Pino-Sedeño, T., Trujillo-Martín, M.M., Andia, I., Aragón-Sánchez, J., Herrera-Ramos, E., Iruzubieta Barragán, F.J., & Serrano-Aguilar, P. (2019). Platelet-rich plasma for the treatment of diabetic foot ulcers: A meta-analysis. *Wound repair and regeneration : official publication of the Wound Healing Society [and] the European Tissue Repair Society,* 27(2), 170-82. Epub 2018 Dec 21. PMID: 30575212 DOI: 10.1111/wrr.12690

# CHAPTER 11:
# PERIPHERAL NEUROPATHY AND
# WOUND HEALING

We were ready for our grand opening for Vampire Facelifts® and Facials®. A dental patient whom I have known for many years, came and learned about PRP. He made an appointment for the next week. I was surprised but delighted. More and more men are getting aesthetic treatments.

At his appointment, he explained that he had Type II Diabetes and that his feet were numb. They felt like they were always asleep with constant pins and needles. He wanted me to inject them with PRP. I told him I could not using my dental license. I am licensed for head and neck only.

He got me thinking though. Would it be a wonderful idea to bring on a medical director? Most medical spas are set up with a medical director and the service providers are nurses or licensed estheticians. The Vampire course included the "O" Shot and the "P" shot which we will go into detail soon.

Where do you find a medical director? It is not like you place a want-ad. But I thought this was a brilliant idea, so I looked for a medical director. My husband and I made a list of the MDs we would ask. I called a few but none were interested. I thought it was a no-brainer. Get paid for no work. The perfect sinecure.

We found one at a party. Yes, you heard that right. I was telling everyone about this exciting thing called PRP. I asked if anyone knew a doctor who wanted to be a medical director. My friend Kathy, an attorney, said, "As a matter of fact, I do." Does he still have a license? Just kidding. He is a good friend of an attorney in her firm.

We met with the doctor and loved him. Such a smart guy. We found a medical director. At last, someone wants a sinecure.

I know I have used the word sinecure two times. Few people know what it means. Here is the back story. One year my husband received a word calendar for Christmas. We planned to expand our vocabulary. Every day we learned an unfamiliar word. At the end of the year, you would think we learned at least a couple hundred words. No, we only remembered one word—sinecure. The definition is that you get paid for no work.

With a medical director, the services we can provide are open to the entire body. The patient that wanted his feet treated didn't come back until six months later. At least, he returned.

When he came in to inject his feet, his pinky toe on his left foot was necrotic. It was black, and the skin was dying. Non-healing diabetic foot ulcers are a common cause of amputation. I told him that I did not know if this would help but I was confident his own plasma would not hurt him. I prayed that it would help because he told me that if he had to have amputations of his lower limbs, he would commit suicide. I believed him and understood his sentiment.

He didn't feel the injections until we were up to his ankles. Usually, we use anesthetic before the PRP injections. He did not need an anesthetic. There was not much feeling in his feet. This is not a good thing.

Less than 15 years ago a research group out of Maryland studied topical use of PRP for chronic ulcers in diabetic patients.[1] They randomized patients into two groups—one group used Platelet Rich Plasma gel the other group used saline gel dressings. Each patient was evaluated biweekly for 12 weeks or until healing. Significantly more Platelet Rich Plasma gel (13 out of 16, 81.3%) healed within the 12 weeks. The patients that used the saline gel healed at a much lower rate than the PRP group. 42.1% compared to 81.3% in the PRP group.

A study published in 2011, followed 285 non-healing skin wounds treated with PRP gel dressing.[2] Diabetes, pressure, or venous ulcer caused the wounds which included dehisced, surgical, or traumatic wounds, and wounds of other etiologies.

They concluded: "In chronic wounds recalcitrant to other treatments, utilization of PRP gel can restart the healing process. Rapid treatment response was observed in 275 of 285 wounds, and the magnitude of response was consistently high, with statistically significant outcomes reported for various subgroups."

This was the last hope for healing.

A study published in 2019 examined the clinical trial database and pulled eight randomized clinical trials.[3] Their conclusion:

1)   treatment with PRP increased the likelihood of chronic wound healing,
2)   ulcer volume decreased
3)   time to complete wound healing decreased

All these wound studies used topical PRP dressings which was effective, however, we injected near the necrotic, diabetic wounds.

This patient with the necrotic black toe called six weeks later. He wanted another injection appointment. On the phone he told me how the black part of that pinky toe had fallen off and it looked better. I couldn't wait to see the toe. Did it get better? There is a reason they call these wounds non-healing because they do not heal.

He walks in the wellness center kicks off his flip flops and proudly shows off his feet.Unfortunately the before and after pictures have been lost but believe me the healing was remarkable in 6 weeks.

The pins and needles feeling in his feet is still very present. The change I noticed was that he felt more of the injections and needed more anesthetic which means feeling is returning to his feet. At least that is the right direction. The patient has not returned to the wellness center but we hope he has avoided amputation for at least a while.

Another patient with diabetes came in for treatment for a diabetic ulcer on the bottom of his big toe. He had already lost his second toe by amputation due to an unresolving ulcer. The treatment before amputation was for the patient to sit in a hyperbaric oxygen tank for 2 ½ hours 5 days a week for 6 weeks. Hyperbaric oxygen therapy increases oxygen availability for the patient by increasing normal air pressure. At that time, he had 2 non-healing ulcers. One toe healed but the other had to be amputated. He was ready to try something different. We injected 5 cc of PRP around the wound. PRP is only a liquid because there is anticoagulant in the test tube. It naturally coagulates. That is its first job—to form a clot. As part of his wound care, we made PRP clots and put them in little jars for him to freeze. He used these clots as part of the wound dressing.

Figure 33: Before PRP treatment

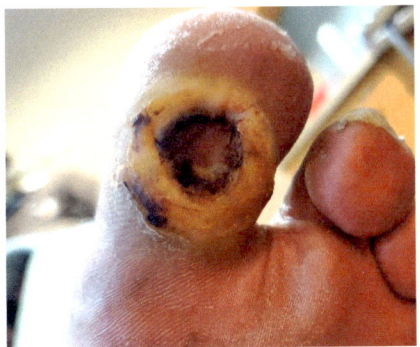

The black seen in the picture is necrotic tissue meaning it is dead skin. The white ring is a callus and the center is the wound area. Notice it is grey. No blood can be seen. The ulcer was about 10 mm across and 15 mm deep.

Figure 34: Before and 2 weeks after the 1st PRP treatment

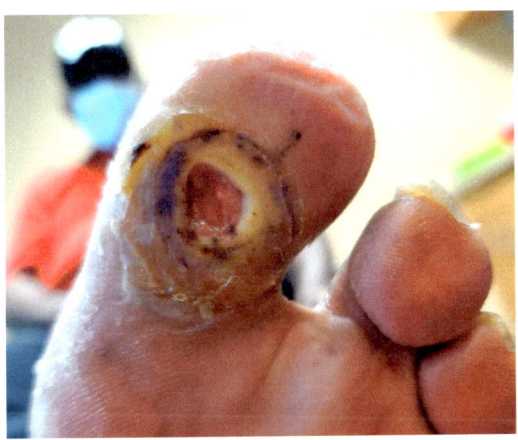

Notice how pink the wound is and the black necrotic tissue is almost gone.

Figure 35: Before, 2 weeks after 1st PRP treatment, 3 weeks after 1st PRP treatment

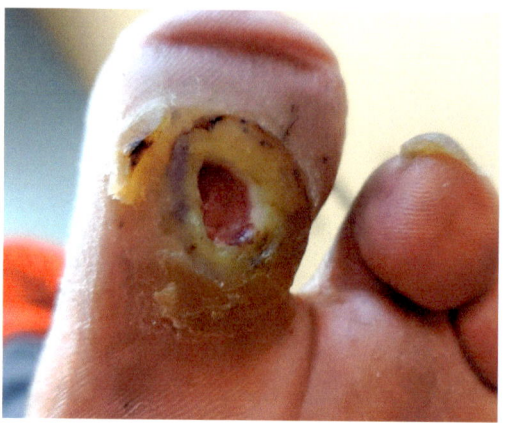

The wound is still pink and is beginning to close. There is less dead tissue and the callus is sloughing away. Unfortunately, this book went to press before we were finished with the treatment, but we will keep you updated on the website www.candcwellness.com.

References for Chapter 11:

1. 1.Miłek, T., Baranowski, K., Zydlewski, P., Ciostek, P., Mlosek, K., & Olszewski, W. (2017). Role of plasma growth factor in the healing of chronic ulcers of the lower legs and foot due to ischaemia in diabetic patients. *Postepy dermatologii i alergologii,* 34(6), 601-6. PMID: 29422826 PMCID: PMC5799748 DOI: 10.5114/pdia.2016.62415

2. 2.de Leon, J.M., Driver, V.R., Fylling, C.P., Carter, M.J., Anderson, C., Wilson, J., ... & Rappl, L.M. (2011). The Clinical Relevance of Treating Chronic Wounds with an Enhanced Near-Physiological Concentration of Platelet-Rich Plasma Gel. *Advances in Skin & Wound Care*, 24(8), 357-68. DOI: 10.1097/01.ASW.0000403249.85131.6f

3. 3.Del Pino-Sedeño, T., Trujillo-Martín, M.M., Andia, I., Aragón-Sánchez, J., Herrera-Ramos, E., Iruzubieta Barragán, F.J., & Serrano-Aguilar, P. (2019). Platelet-rich plasma for the treatment of diabetic foot ulcers: A meta-analysis. *Wound repair and regeneration : official publication of the Wound Healing Society [and] the European Tissue Repair Society,* 27(2), 170-82. Epub 2018 Dec 21. PMID: 30575212 DOI: 10.1111/wrr.12690

# CHAPTER 12:
# ARTHRITIS

There are two studies that have examined PRP and wrist/thumb arthritis. One study compared corticosteroids to PRP at three months and then again at 12 months.[1] The steroids gave short-term relief, however the PRP gave significant long-term relief at 12 months.

The other study followed 10 patients that received PRP injection at three months and six months and concluded that PRP is a reasonable therapy with good outcomes and very safe.[2] All studies end with stating there needs to be another study. They are in the business of producing papers and conducting studies.

There are many studies looking at osteoarthritis of the knee. There are similar outcomes of reduced pain at 12 months. One study compared one PRP injection versus multiple injections and concluded that multiple injections had more benefit.[3] Both single injection and multile injections improved pain management, however, multiple injections improved joint functionality which led to an improved lifestyle.

Physicians and therapists have used PRP in orthopedic/sports medicine for a long time. Many patients report that their doctors offer PRP for rotator cuff surgery, for example.

My observation is rapid healing of any area where we inject PRP. I would not have surgery without demanding PRP over a surgical area before closing and the outside of the sutures. There is a medical device that is like a little gun. It shoots PRP and calcium chloride and thrombin into the surgical site. The calcium chloride and thrombin cause the PRP to clot, and "stick it" to the area. The PRP stays in the surgical area and begins the healing process. This is what the body would naturally send to the surgical area. This jump starts rapid healing.

In our dental office, we have a surgeon who removes 3rd molars, and he started using PRP in the socket and infiltrating the area with liquid PRP. The first stage of healing is clotting. If we add no anticoagulant to the test tube, the PRP forms a yellow gel ball. He takes that gel ball and places it in the socket and sutures it in. Then the liquid PRP is injected next to the socket. The healing and recovery from wisdom tooth extraction has been phenomenal. We want our patients to have the best recovery possible and we have found it. The patient is still sore the first couple of days as the healing gets started, but the healing time is reduced and there are not any dry sockets. A dry socket is when the patient loses the natural clot from the extraction site. It is a painful condition because it exposes the bone to the environment. With the PRP gel ball in the socket, it is a natural band-aid or a healing dressing. It traps all those beautiful healing factors in for the duration of the healing process.

At the post-op check, the patients report that they did not need the pain medication at all, and the extraction sites are beautifully healed..

References for Chapter 12:

1.  Forogh, B., Mianehsaz, E., Shoaee, S., Ahadi, T., Raissi, G.R., & Sajadi, S. (2016). Effect of single injection of platelet-rich plasma in comparison with corticosteroid on knee osteoarthritis: a double-blind randomized clinical trial. *The Journal of sports medicine and physical fitness,* 56(7-8), 901-8. Epub 2015 Jul 14. PMID: 26173792

2.  Loibl, M., Lang, S., Dendl, L., Nerlich, M., Angele, P., Gehmert, S., & Huber, M. (2016). Leukocyte-Reduced Platelet-Rich Plasma Treatment of Basal Thumb Arthritis: A Pilot Study. *BioMed Research International*, 2016, 1-6. DOI: 10.1155/2016/9262909

3.  Tavassoli, M., Janmohammadi, N., Hosseini, A., Khafri, S., & Esmaeilnejad-Ganji, S.M. (2019). Single- and double-dose of platelet-rich plasma versus hyaluronic acid for treatment of knee osteoarthritis: A randomized controlled trial. *World journal of orthopedics,* 10(9), 310-26. PMID: 31572668 PMCID: PMC6766465 DOI: 10.5312/wjo.v10.i9.310

# CHAPTER 13:
# TEETH

My patient, Gloria, had a tooth that had bothered her for over a year. On and off hot and cold sensitivity, and she had biting pressure which made it difficult to eat. The tooth did not cause her severe pain but a constant dull pain and constant annoyance. I understand why other medical providers do not think to use something new in their practices. They are too close to think outside the box. My dental assistant had to suggest injecting PRP next to the tooth. SHAZAM! Why didn't I think of that?

I numbed the area, drew blood, ran it through the centrifuge and injected next to the affected tooth, crossed my fingers and said a prayer. But why wouldn't it help heal a tooth? It healed a toenail, a tendon, a scar, a necrotic wound, etc. We have used PRP in dentistry for over 30 years but only for bone grafts, never for hurt teeth.

A few days after the PRP treatment, I reached out to see if the tooth was any better. This is Gloria's answer, "I'm cautiously optimistic. There seems to be less sensitivity and pain. However, the tooth still 'flares up' throughout the day. I want to make sure that there is not a placebo effect; however, I think it is better. I am hoping it will continue to improve. It just seems slow, but I'll take it."

Fantastic! It is a wait and see game.

About a month later, I got an update: "I can for certain say that I no longer have constant pain in my tooth. There is still sensitivity to hot and cold and some pressure but nothing like the pain I was experiencing. I hope that the sensitivity will decrease over time."

Teeth do not heal easily or quickly. There is little blood flow. The nerve lives in the tooth's root which is a hard box that does not give. Unlike other areas in your body, if there is swelling in a tooth there is no place for the nerve to go. It hits the sides of the root.

PRP opens a whole new way to treat upset teeth but maybe not when they are infected. But PRP is antimicrobial, so maybe a study treating infected teeth is my next project. Maybe patients do not need a root canal. They may need tender loving healing.

I am happy to report that Gloria's tooth is no longer causing pain three months after one PRP treatment, but she still has some sensitivity. As she says, "nothing unlivable." I suggested we do another injection. She agreed.

References for Chapter 13:

1. Li, H., & Li, B. (2013). PRP as a new approach to prevent infection: preparation and in vitro antimicrobial properties of PRP. *Journal of visualized experiments :* J Vis Exp 2013 Apr 9; (74):50351    DOI: 10.3791/50351 PMID:23609458

# CHAPTER 14:
# O–SHOT

At the Vampire course, we also learned how to give the O-shot. If you haven't heard of it, you will. It is injecting PRP into the vagina and clitoris. Before you yell, "Ouch, NO WAY!" Hear me out.

The PRP does the same thing for the vaginal skin as it does for your face skin. It creates new mucosa, increases blood vessels and collagen. It provides all aspects of healing. This healing then improves orgasm because new nerve connections increase sensitivity.

The vagina is the only organ whose sole purpose is to produce pleasure. As we age, we lose the bounce to create that pleasure. We get drier and drier. Sexual intercourse becomes painful. As my grandmother used to say, "Growing older isn't for wimps." We have a magnificent tool to ease the symptoms of aging, PRP. It is natural, and it is your own healing factors. All we do is concentrate it in a specific body part including the vagina.

The O-shot improves urinary incontinence. Many women (and men but they don't talk about it) have leaky bladders. We can't jump or laugh or sneeze or run without peeing on ourselves. A good friend of mine said she was so sick of having to wear a pad everyday all day, she had to at least try the O-shot. She loves it. In one month, she has stopped peeing on herself. She is healing.

You know those ads for the incontinent panties. Did you see where they added a little butterfly to the panties? Is that supposed to make it better? You still peed in your pants. I am sorry, urine has an odor and needs to be disposed of in the toilet. There is a better solution than accepting having to wear diapers for the rest of your adult-life.

Let me address the elephant in the room. How much does it hurt? It does NOT hurt, and I will tell you why: Great numbing cream and ice. The mucosa (skin) is like the gums in the mouth. It absorbs the numbing cream. You get really numb from the cream.

Have you ever seen the big square whiskey ice cubes? They are 1 ½ inches square and are easy to hold. We wrap a paper towel around the ice cube and you hold it down there until it feels really cold. Between the numbing cream, the Lidocaine and the ice, you don't feel anything but pressure. We then inject the PRP into the vaginal wall and the clitoris.

The first time I got the O-shot was at Dr. Runels course in front of 10 doctors and nurses, but I had to live it so I could tell my patients about the experience. It was well worth it. I promise it did NOT hurt. It was pressure. Period.

This is such a life changing procedure. It is non-invasive, safe and effective. And look at the benefits!

We have observed that all we have to do is get the PRP near the damaged tissue. It will go where it needs to go. Heal what it needs to heal. I read one study where researchers talked about directing PRP and told it what to do. Man will tell God what to do? No way! PRP is the healing that God created in each one of us. Man will just screw it up.

A long timedental patient came down to the new wellness center to see what we were up to. We talked about all the services we provide. She stopped us to ask all about the O-shot. It turns out they had diagnosed her with lichen sclerosus. The gynecologist had given her steroid cream which had not helped at all. She was in great discomfort and wanted to know if the O-shot would help that condition.

Lichen sclerosus can appear on any part of the body but prefers the genital area. In Wikipedia, it states, "In adults, LS is incurable, and often gets worse." It appears as white plaques and raw skin. It is not painful in the beginning but as the condition continues to get worse, it can become painful.

She was desperate and wanted to at least try the O-shot. I found several studies that showed promising results. When we treated her, I almost cried at the condition of her skin. It had white plaques, but it was raw with open wounds. I am happy to report that at her 6-week checkup, she was 95% healed. We did a second O-shot, and she is 100% healed. She continues to feel great.

**P-Shot (Priapus Shot)**

You are correct. Is this for males? Yes. What is Priapus? It is a "who." Priapus is the Greek God of Lust. Look him up. Dr. Runels is an intelligent, educated man and I know he thought this was funny. It is hilarious.

When I came back from the Vampire course, I told my young male associate, Dr. Dave, "I went to this course and learned how to do the Vampire Facelift® and the Vampire Facial®. We also learned about the P-Shot." He asked, "What's that?" When I explained the P-Shot his face turned white then red. He was aghast. I said, "Wait until it doesn't work then you will understand."

The P-shot helps with improving erections and urinary incontinence which is common after prostate surgery. Nobody enjoys peeing in their pants. I don't care how old you are or if you are male or female.

The immune cells in PRP are antibacterial and have immune properties. A study looking at these properties found that PRP was bactericidal for gonorrhoeae in the genital tract. There is so much more to learn [1].

The same numbing cream we use on the vaginal tissue is used to numb the penis, and it really works. Dentists use an anesthetic called Septocaine that numbs quickly and profoundly. We use that instead of Lidocaine. You may never convince your mate to get a P-Shot but at least you know about it, especially for urinary incontinence if it ever becomes a problem.

References for Chapter 14:

1. 1.Li, H., & Li, B. (2013). PRP as a new approach to prevent infection: preparation and in vitro antimicrobial properties of PRP. *Journal of visualized experiments: JoVE,* PMID:23609458 PMCID:PMC3653398 DOI:10.3791/50351

# CHAPTER 15:
# ANTIBACTERIAL PROPERTIES OF PRP

A s you know, PRP is known for its ability to clot a wound but who would have guessed the fantastic antibacterial properties. Most of the attention has been on bone grafting, injury repair (tendons and ligaments) and regeneration (Vampire Facial®) while the anti-infectious advantages have been overlooked.

In 2000, researchers published a study looking at the non-hemostatic functions, in other words, functions that have nothing to do with blood clotting.[1] There are at least three functions: inflammation, immunity and tissue repair. As primary immune cells, platelets contain microbicidal proteins that kill bacteria within five minutes in a petri dish. There are also anti-fungal proteins capable of wiping out fungal infections

In a recent study, they examined tissue infections and bone infections and using PRP as an adjunct to standard treatments of debridement and antibiotics the results were outstanding [2]. This is a repetitive story. Everything PRP touches heals and why not? It is the system God set up to heal ourselves.

Researchers published one of the most remarkable examples of the immune function in *Science*, when platelets killed malarial organisms within infected red blood cells [3].

I was thinking about PRP because I am obsessed and think about it all the time. I thought, of course it has antibacterial properties. It had to for our protection. It probably has anti-viral properties. No one has looked yet. God knew you would skin your knee, wipe off the blood and keep playing. Who has time to go home to Mommy? There had to be protection from the natural enemies, bacteria and everything else. We have built in defenses against them. It only makes sense.

One of the most interesting hypotheses is can PRP be effective antimicrobial against the potentially fatal drug-resistant infections? MRSA (Methicillin Resistant Staphylococcus Aureus) is one of the leading causes of hospital-acquired and post-operative infections. MRSA is the bacteria that is resistant to ALL antibiotics. They are super bugs.

In a study, they divided six lab animals into two groups. A full-thickness skin wound was created then a MRSA (Methicillin Resistant Staphylococcus Aureus) suspension was injected into the wound [4]. One group received PRP and the other group received conventional debridement and antibiotics.

Treatment started 1-week post introduction of the infection and wound creation. The PRP group received subcutaneous PRP every week. The control group received a topical application of the antibiotic clindamycin twice daily.

The study compared standard protocols for wound care of debridement and antibiotics to debridement and PRP. You guessed it. The PRP did better with healing and killing the infection. I know what you are thinking, "Why isn't the medical industry using PRP for these especially impossible situations?" The answer lies in the reality of life. Everyone is busy. We cannot expect the physician to go home and start reading studies. He or she has a family and obligations. This is new in the medical world. You may not think 30 years is new, but medical practitioners are waiting for it to be examined under laboratory conditions. Like I said before, we have used it in dentistry, orthopedics and equine medicine out of necessity. In dentistry, the bone graft did not take well without PRP. In orthopedics, tendons and ligaments do not heal quickly or at all. In equine medicine, horses are just worth a lot of money! I joke that if you want the best medicine follow the practices in veterinary medicine, especially horse medicine.

I had my husband inject my left knee because it was a little tweaky. It wasn't anything to go to the doctor for; however, it bothered me during yoga. He injected my knee all around and it healed. About three weeks later, I realized the knee stopped bothering me but now I felt tweaky in the right knee. Glenna, my nurse, injected the right knee but this time I had one injection in the meaty muscle above the knee. It healed in about three weeks.

Here is a paradigm shift. Because PRP has great antibacterial properties, they could use it in surgery before closing and on the sutures and one could not need systemic antibiotics. PRP also has anti-inflammatory mechanisms that would reduce the need for pain meds. If the patient healed up twice as fast, there would be less down time. All good properties don't you agree? Until it becomes mainstream, most physicians will not even offer patients the choice of receiving PRP as an adjunct to a surgery. But as the patient, you can ask for PRP. What is the worst-case scenario? They say, "No." What most offices will tell you is that your insurance will not pay for it. I recommend you pay for it. What I have seen is remarkable. It is well worth healing more easily and more quickly.

References for Chapter 15:

1. 1.Krijgsveld, J., Zaat, S.A., Meeldijk, J., van Veelen, P.A., Fang, G., Poolman, B., ... & Dankert, J. (2000). Thrombocidins, microbicidal proteins from human blood platelets, are C-terminal deletion products of CXC chemokines. *The Journal of biological chemistry,* 275(27), 20374-81. PMID: 10877842 DOI: 10.1074/jbc.275.27.20374

2. 2.Zhang, W., Guo, Y., Kuss, M., Shi, W., Aldrich, A.L., Untrauer, J., ... & Duan, B. (2019). Platelet-Rich Plasma for the Treatment of Tissue Infection: Preparation and Clinical Evaluation. *Tissue Engineering Part B: Reviews*, 25(3), 225-36. DOI:10.1089/ten.TEB.2018.0309

3. 3.McMorran BJ, Marshall VM, de Graaf C, Drysdale KE, Shabbar M, Smyth GK, Corbin JE, Alexander WS, Foote SJ, (2009) Platelets kill intraerythrocytic malarial parasites and mediate survival to infection. Science 323(5915):797-800. DOI:10.1126/science.1166296

4. 4.Farghali, H.A., AbdElKader, N.A., AbuBakr, H.O., Aljuaydi, S.H., Khattab, M.S., Elhelw, R., & Elhariri, M. (2019). Antimicrobial action of autologous platelet-rich plasma on MRSA-infected skin wounds in dogs. *Scientific reports,* 9(1), 12722. DOI: 10.1038/s41598-019-48657-5. PMID:31481694

# CHAPTER 16:
# SHINGLES AND PLANTA FASCIITIS

I have two stories about shingles and PRP. The herpes zoster virus causes shingles that flares up later in life. Chicken pox also comes from the same virus.

Shingles is a painful rash with excruciating shooting pain. It shows up on one side of your body and the shooting pain can remain as skin sensitivity for years.

One doctor at the Vampire course received PRP on his head for hair regrowth to improve male pattern baldness. The next day at lunch he announced he had shingles about one year before the course and since that outbreak he could not sleep on his right side. The skin on the right side of his head was too sensitive to put pressure on the area. After he received PRP injections for balding, he could sleep on his right side that night! He didn't have any sensitivity. It sounds crazy that it can have an instant effect, but we have observed other instantaneous nerve responses. We saw nerve response this quickly with the patient with Bell's palsy. The other observation is that some conditions treated with PRP take weeks to see improvement and multiple treatments. Some symptoms improve right away. Other symptoms improve within a few weeks.

The other patient with shingles had an active shingle outbreak on her back. There is a limited number of successful treatments for shingles. Most treatments are palliative. We injected the area around the outbreak with shingles and it calmed down quickly.

Shingles breaks out with stress and this patient is under extreme stress. A second outbreak occurred about three months later. Another PRP treatment was necessary, and it erased all the signs or symptoms of shingles.

**Plantar Fasciitis**

My sister, Marian, came to the office for a Vampire Facelift® and casually mentioned her doctor diagnosed her with plantar fasciitis. She experienced pain every morning when she first put weight on the right foot. It worked itself out as the day went on, but the pain was back the next morning.

As Wikipedia describes, plantar fasciitis is a disorder involving the connective tissue which supports the arch of the foot. The most common clinical presentation is heel pain; however, pain often takes place elsewhere in the foot. The research shows that this condition involves very little inflammation as the name would imply. Instead, it is a degenerative process of micro tears and degeneration of collagen in the ligaments and tendons. There is also evidence of fascial thickening. Fascia is tendon-like fibrous connective tissue that runs throughout our bodies forming compartments, for example, surrounding muscles and organs. It is like cellophane running throughout the body keeping organs and other structures contained.

The researchers concluded in several studies that when compared to corticosteroid injection, PRP had a better outcome at 12 months.[1][2] These studies showed that the steroid injection may reduce pain quicker at first but that the patients had less pain and better function at the 12month follow up appointment.

This has been a magnificent year of discovery and learning. Watching patients heal quickly is rewarding. Everyone needs to know PRP is a viable treatment for many ailments. PRP is full of glorious healing factors that are ready to work for you.

It seems modern medicine has put itself into a non-thinking box. Everything has become an algorithm. The dictionary defines an algorithm as "a step-by-step procedure for solving a problem or accomplishing some end." The powers-that-be setup step-by-step medicine to make medicine more uniform and logical. The problem is that once they write an algorithm, there is no reward for thinking outside the box. In fact, they discourage physicians from coming at a problem from a different direction.

It also seems that once someone writes the algorithm, and it is and adopted, it never changes. Fresh ideas are not tried. Anyone with a novel idea, must run a double-blind placebo-controlled study and many times this is impossible and expensive. Case studies and clinical observations are legitimate science.

Have you noticed that whenever you go to the doctor with a pain symptom of any kind the answer is always a steroid shot or steroid pack? It is the algorithm for pain. As we discussed earlier, the reason you can only have three injections in one area is because steroids stop the healing process and destruction of the area ensues.

Maybe a better answer is to heal the problem-not mask the pain. The key is getting a proper diagnosis and being smart about your treatment options. PRP is you healing you!

I filled this book with clinical observations that have been impressive. I had to share them with everyone. We started with the esthetic side of

PRP with the Vampire Facial and found changes that were phenomenal. Patients tell us they feel much better about themselves every time they look in the mirror. They love having smaller pores and the vibrant glow one cannot get from anything else on the market.

My friend has a new grandbaby and her daughter posted a picture of grandma and baby on Facebook. One of the posted comments stated, "You must love being a grandmother; you are glowing!" She loves being a grandma, but there were also three PRP treatments!

Seeing a severe scar heal and disappear is spectacular. Scars do not disappear within 12 weeks. If they disappear at all, it is because many years have passed. We keep learning and are amazed at the properties of PRP. Stay connected. I write a blog and I regularly update it. The blog is on our website candcwellness.com or look for us on Facebook.

It is an exciting time to think you always had the power to heal yourself and you can use those healing properties in smart ways. PRP is YOU HEALING YOU!

References for Chapter 16:

1.  Shetty, S.H., Dhond, A., Arora, M., & Deore, S. (2019). Platelet-Rich Plasma Has Better Long-Term Results Than Corticosteroids or Placebo for Chronic Plantar Fasciitis: Randomized Control Trial. *The Journal of foot and ankle surgery : official publication of the American College of Foot and Ankle Surgeons,* 58(1), 42-6. PMID: 30448183 DOI: 10.1053/j.jfas.2018.07.006

2.  Peerbooms, J.C., Lodder, P., den Oudsten, B.L., Doorgeest, K., Schuller, H.M., & Gosens, T. (2019). Positive Effect of Platelet-Rich Plasma on Pain in Plantar Fasciitis: A Double-Blind Multicenter Randomized Controlled Trial. *The American journal of sports medicine,* 47(13), 3238-46. DOI: 10.1177/0363546519877181 PMID: 31603721

# FREQUENTLY ASKED QUESTION

**What are PRP injections?**

Platelet Rich Plasma injections is based on the idea that we use the body's natural healing method and concentrate this natural healing in an injured area. The Platelet Rich Plasma or PRP for short is an element of everyone's blood. We draw blood in test tubes and spin in a centrifuge. The blood separates into 2 fractions. Red blood cells are heavier than plasma and thereby fall to the bottom of the test tube. PRP floats on top of the red blood cells and is easily removed. PRP contains the healing factors called growth factors. We inject those healing factors into an injured area concentrating natural healing where it is needed. The number of injections needed depends on the diagnosis and the nature of the injury.

**Why use PRP injections?**

We use PRP injections when the patient wants an effective treatment alternative. It is used to speed up healing after surgery or as an alternative to surgery especially for muscle strains and ligament or tendon injuries.

We also use it as an esthetic treatment in the Vampire Facial. The healing factors heal aging skin building collagen, smoothing wrinkles and decreasing pore size, to name a few.

**How does PRP work?**

PRP contains many healing factors. When it is injected at the site of injury, the healing factors are concentrated in that area. These healing factors (growth factors) initiate healing by inducing the healing chemical cascade in the same way your body naturally heals a skinned knee with PRP. PRP will heal tendons, muscles, skin, blood vessels, build collagen and cartilage. Given enough time the body will heal. The injections speed up the recovery rate.

**What are PRP side effects?**

The side effects include some soreness at the injection site. PRP induces the inflammatory response as it is the first step of the healing chemical cascade. There may be some swelling and soreness during the first 48 hours. Most patients do not need pain medication during the first 2 days post injection.

**How quickly does PRP work?**

Depending on the injury, most patients see improvement within 2 – 6 weeks. Many patients see much better long-term improvements with PRP injections than with steroid injections. PRP is a healing modality and not a quick pain relief treatment. The pain relief comes as the injured tissue heals which takes weeks or months.

The facial rejuvenation begins immediately and continues to enhance beauty for 8 to 12 weeks.

**Are PRP injections safe?**

PRP injections are very safe. There are no foreign substances being injected. It is your own blood being injected back into you. There is no possibility of rejection because it is your own plasma.

This method has been used for many years in a few medical fields including dentistry, equine medicine, and orthopedics. As our knowledge grows, the uses for PRP are expanding.

**Is there any patient who would not be a good candidate for PRP?**

If a patient has a blood disorder, it is not recommended to use PRP. These conditions include low platelet count, abnormal platelet function, severe anemia, and systemic infection.

**Is PRP injection therapy right for me?**

As with all medical conditions, diagnosis is the key. With the right diagnosis, PRP is effective treatment for many conditions. Many patients are searching for an alternative to surgery and PRP is a good option.

# ABOUT THE AUTHOR

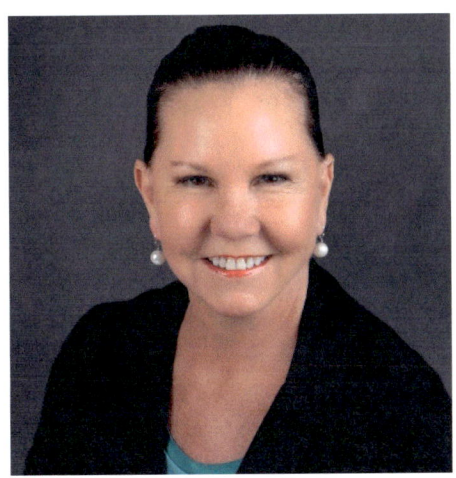

Prior to moving to Houston, Texas as a young teenager, Dr. Teresa Cody lived with her family in Brussels, Belgium. She earned her undergraduate degree at the University of Texas at Austin, then her Doctor of Dental Surgery at the University of Texas Dental Branch in Houston in 1992. The next year she and her new husband, also a dentist, bought a practice in Sugar Land, TX. They routinely used PRP therapy to promote healing after bone graft surgery, so she knew the Platelet Rich Plasma injections were effective.

During a routine visit to her hair dresser, she suggested using the therapy to address the damage done to her hair dresser's hand after nearly forty years of repetitive motions in the beauty salon. The woman couldn't touch her fingers with her thumb. Within twelve hours after the injection, she could again touch her thumb to her fingers. Within two days she could make a fist. Dr. Cody realized she's discovered a powerful response to such diverse health challenges as aging skin issues, Bell's Palsy, clearing up ugly scars and giving relief to joint pain.

In February 2019 Dr. Cody opened the C and C Wellness Center, where the incredible results she witnessed inspired her to write *You Healing You.* She wrote the book to introduce others to the multiple health benefits of PRP treatments. Dr. Cody focuses her energy on research studies using PRP, as well as, writing and speaking to spread the information about the benefits of Platelet Rich Plasma injections.

Made in the USA
Columbia, SC
21 August 2024

40609062R00062